LIFE SUPPORT

MIKE RUBIN

LIFE SUPP⬥RT

ENTERTAINMENT, ADVICE, AND ENCOURAGEMENT
FOR FIRST RESPONDERS

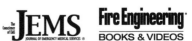

Disclaimer

The recommendations, advice, descriptions, and methods in this book are presented solely for educational purposes. The author and publisher assume no liability whatsoever for any loss or damage that results from the use of any of the material in this book. Use of the material in this book is solely at the risk of the user.

Copyright © 2021 by
Fire Engineering Books & Videos
110 S. Hartford Ave., Suite 200
Tulsa, Oklahoma 74120 USA

800.752.9764
+1.918.831.9421
info@fireengineeringbooks.com
www.FireEngineeringBooks.com

Senior Vice President: Eric Schlett
Operations Manager: Holly Fournier
Sales Manager: Joshua Neal
Managing Editor: Mark Haugh
Production Manager: Tony Quinn
Developmental Editor: Chris Barton
Book Designer: Robert Kern, TIPS Technical Publishing, Inc., Carrboro, NC
Cover Designer: Trent Farar
Cover photo courtesy of Steve Silverman

Library of Congress Cataloging-in-Publication Data

Names: Rubin, Mike, 1953- author.
Title: Life support : entertainment, advice, and encouragement for first
    responders / Mike Rubin.
Description: Tulsa, Oklahoma : Fire Engineering Books and Videos, [2021] |
    Includes index. | Summary: "A compilation of educational and humorous
    essays for first responders by EMS Today magazine contributor Michael
    Rubin. Topics covered include career advice, personal growth, and
    patient care"-- Provided by publisher.
Identifiers: LCCN 2021034419 | ISBN 9781593705756 (trade paperback)
Subjects: LCSH: First responders--United States--Anecdotes. | Emergency
    management--United States--Anecdotes.
Classification: LCC HV554.3 .R83 2021 | DDC 362.180973--dc23
LC record available at https://lccn.loc.gov/2021034419

Printed in the United States of America

1 2 3 4 5   25 24 23 22 21

To Helen,
who cares for the caregivers.

CONTENTS

News and Views

In Case You're Interested . . .

INTRODUCTION

The summer of 2018 was EMS refresher time for me. I needed to renew my ACLS and PALS certifications as part of my paramedic CME. I don't mind learning stuff, but the prospect of spending four days on mind-numbing repeats of 2016 AHA curricula made me want to text both instructors the same excuse about the dog eating my algorithms. I might have if my wife hadn't intervened.

"You have to go," Helen said.

"Yeah, because I need those hours."

"No, because I invited the girls over for lunch."

Oh.

Why fuss over a few days in the company of manikins? Because I hate being tested on anything. I've felt that way since I had to memorize the capitals of all 48 states when I was five—my mother's idea. She said it would make me smart like Albert Einstein, but it only made me neurotic like Woody Allen.

Megacodes are my least favorite exams. They're almost always too contrived to be realistic. When your patients are mute, polyurethane torsos and you have neither visual cues nor functioning diagnostic equipment, those scenarios usually devolve into strained dialogues and predictable outcomes.

"What do I see?" I always ask the preceptor about imaginary patients.

"Like what, for example?"

"Like everything—the scene, the patient's affect, the skin, fluids, signs of distress."

"The scene is safe," I'm invariably told, as if danger could be willed away. "The patient's unresponsive. You notice difficulty breathing, a hole in the right chest, and tracheal shift."

If only EMS were that easy.

I've written several articles about the futility of script-driven simulation, and find Q&A with bored examiners hard to take seriously.

Yet I still needed ACLS and PALS cards. No amount of complaining was going to change that.

Being from the proactive branch of my family, I pitched short, first-person pieces about those alphabet courses to Jon, my editor at *EMS World*. I assumed AHA refreshers would be easier to tolerate as a writer than a paramedic.

Jon understands the limits of tedious oral exams. I say that because he's never asked me to prove I speak English by reciting all the synonyms for tedious. Thank you, Jon. You're an awesome editor, but I doubt you have a future as an ACLS instructor.

Jon and I decided I'd attend hospital-based ACLS and PALS programs and report on my experiences. I figured the promise of paying gigs would force me to show up, thereby satisfying some prerequisites for my 2019 paramedic license. You'll find reviews of those classes under "ACLS 2018: Did You Hear the One About the Medic and the ABG?" and "PALS 2018: Hooked On Mnemonics."

While writing those commentaries, I recalled other playful pieces I'd authored for *EMS World's* magazine as part of our monthly Life Support series from 2009 through 2015. I browsed those columns and found most of them as timely as when they'd first appeared. Their topics—loyalty, safety, compassion, competence, etc.—are lighter and less technical than most of what you've read about EMS in textbooks and periodicals. I started to think some of that material might be worth reissuing.

Next, I looked at my more educational contributions to *EMS World*. Some were outdated, but most—features on patient assessment, finances, negotiation, and job interviews, for example—were still current. Why not add them to the mix?

After weeding out less-compelling items, I had 80 articles I thought would appeal not only to a new audience, but also to long-time readers, many of whom had enjoyed those stories the first time around. I added new material to some chapters, re-edited all of them, and named the compilation *Life Support*, after my former column. I think that title speaks to the book's empathy for caregivers and relevance to EMS.

What I needed next was a publisher. That turned out to be Fire Engineering Books & Videos, who shared my vision and helped make a decent idea better. Together, we polished this collection of EMS essays and presented it in two parts: one for short, light, mostly entertaining content ("News and Views") and the other for educational but not overly technical topics ("In Case You're Interested . . .").

I hope you find both sections worthwhile. Feel free to skip around. And thanks for giving *Life Support* a chance.

NEWS AND VIEWS

LIGHTS, CAMERA, LUNACY!
EMS IN THE MOVIES

2010

Big-screen EMS fiction is just that: fiction. A totally realistic movie about EMS probably wouldn't get past the initial sales pitch, because most of what we do is about as exciting as changing batteries.

If I'd ever found an employer, medical director, and legislature that allowed me to try half of what movie medics do, I would have dropped anchor in that town and spent my workdays yelling things like, "I don't care what the book says; you better hand me that rib spreader before I hit you with this Halligan tool." (Memo to EMS filmmakers: You can use that line if you promise to let me direct the airborne lung-transplant scene.)

Despite a credibility gap wider than Montana, EMS movies can be entertaining when accompanied by a willing suspension of disbelief. At least that's what I tell myself each time I see some clueless actor rubbing defibrillator paddles together. I decided to pursue the notion of prehospital care as cinéma vérité by watching six rescue-oriented films, then offering commentary from an EMS perspective. Just a few ground rules about the format before we begin:

• Ratings are 0-4 stars according to my admittedly biased concept of entertainment: Four stars would be a *Godfather* prequel where Michael Corleone becomes a made paramedic. Zero stars would be a home video of me lip-synching "It's Five O'clock Somewhere."

- One of the reasons EMS people watch EMS movies is to ridicule inaccuracies. We consider it our duty to educate non-EMS viewers, many of whom will never again accept invitations to our homes. *Voodoo EMS* previews scenes you might want to interrupt with snide remarks.
- Segments headed *Say Again?* show dialogue you probably wouldn't hear anywhere except on a movie set. I think you'll find these lines funny, although some aren't supposed to be.

The beer is cold, the popcorn's hot, the kids are in the tool shed—it's showtime!

Broken Vessels (1998)

Rating: *

Plot summary

Tom, who must be the only Penn graduate in history to settle for EMT certification instead of a degree, is hired by "L.A. City Rescue" as a partner for Jimmy, a veteran paramedic who passed burnout long ago and is headed for meltdown. We get the impression Jimmy knows something about medicine when he resuscitates a traumatic arrest and clears another patient's obstructed airway. On the same call. (Memo to the producers: I try to break the monotony of traumatic arrests and obstructed airways by delivering premature twins on even-numbered days.)

Mostly, though, Jimmy does drugs. Then he steals from patients to do even more drugs. When Tom follows his lead, the result is a soulless, mutually destructive partnership that makes Leopold and Loeb look like The Sunshine Boys. Whenever you think it can't get worse, Tom and Jimmy commit another felony, then justify the outcome by babbling us-against-the-world rhetoric. All of this made me want to send Christmas cards to even my most incorrigible partners.

Will Tom plunge ever deeper into Jimmy's nether world, or will he seek salvation after realizing he's the poster child for poor impulse control? Yes.

Voodoo EMS

- When the guys respond to their first call as partners, Jimmy distracts a sword-swinging maniac just before a police officer tackles the wacko through an open window. I'm sure they practice that at the academy. Then Jimmy subdues the EDP with a trans-trousers shot of an unnamed tranquilizer. Didn't I see that on *Animal Planet*? Without the trousers, I mean.
- When a docile patient takes offense at Jimmy's offer of a "beatdown," Jimmy wields a defibrillator as a stun gun, using classic temporal-temporal paddle placement. I think I had a partner who tried that once. On himself.

Say again?

- *"I can't believe I didn't check his air passage."*—Tom, experiencing turbulent *thought* passage.
- *"So, you prefer the high-action calls?"*—Tom to Jimmy, sounding like a mixture of Starsky, Hutch, and Liberace.
- *"Coronary! We have a massive heart attack."*—Tom, just as an elderly patient clutches his chest—you know, like they always do.
- *"What's it like to do heroin?"*—Tom to Jimmy, getting a head-start on CME.

Subjective assessment

Broken Vessels is no more an EMS movie than *Apocalypse Now* is a war movie. My concern is whether the non-EMS audience understands that. Probably not, which is why I'm glad this flick was seen by maybe 83 people, half of whom are related to the cast or crew.

This is a film about drug addiction—about reaching bottom and the consequences of irresponsibility. There's nothing noble about Tom and Jimmy. They don't deserve our sympathy. If you feel the least bit nostalgic while watching the EMS scenes, shred your card right now. Please. Or send it to me and I'll do it for you.

On the lighter side, there's a marvelous performance by Susan Traylor as Suzy, a quirky, hyperactive neighbor whose eccentricities are chemical in origin. Her fate demonstrates that even adorable drug addicts can be dangerous.

Bringing Out the Dead (1999)

Rating: * * *

Plot summary

Frank Pierce is one messed-up paramedic. He works the night shift at fictional Our Lady of Perpetual Mercy hospital in New York's Hell's Kitchen of the early '90s. He's still got game—in the opening scene he intubates a cardiac arrest victim and starts an IV in less time than it takes his partner to attach electrodes—but he's haunted by memories of an 18-year-old asthmatic named Rose who died under his care.

Frank routinely calls in sick or shows up late for work, hoping he'll be dismissed and his torment will end. Instead of discipline, though, his supervisor substitutes sympathy, then cites manpower shortages and sends Frank back to the streets with a promise he'll be fired tomorrow. But there are no tomorrows for Frank—just one joyless shift after another with partners like Larry, preoccupied by the timing and pedigree of his next meal, and Marcus, who's so burnt he's not allowed to work two nights in a row.

As Frank, Nicolas Cage has just the right blend of intensity and vulnerability. John Goodman, Ving Rhames, and Tom Sizemore give credible performances as Frank's erratic partners. My favorite character, though, was the supervisor who barks like a dog in mid-sentence. I'm pretty sure I rode with him. Seriously.

Voodoo EMS

On-duty drinking, abuse of patients, suicidal driving, and other madness portray a system and city out of control. The carnage will make you cringe more than chuckle. The movie is even scarier if you consider that the non-stop procedural aberrancies, while exaggerated, are based on real-life aspects of NYC*EMS in the 80s and early 90s.

Say again?

The funniest lines in this movie are delivered by an unseen dispatcher, played by director Martin Scorsese, who sends crews to:

- A man hearing celebrity voices
- An elderly woman abducted by her cat

- A demonic possession
- A man who set his pants on fire
- A three-car accident—"two taxis and a taxi"
- A man with a noose around his neck and nothing to hang it on
- Fired workers shooting each other at the post office

Subjective assessment

When I first saw this movie 10 years ago, I found it disturbing and depressing. After eight years in EMS, the last thing I wanted was to spend my downtime watching composite replays of the scariest scenes, worst hospitals, and most difficult cases I'd encountered.

I still think *Bringing Out the Dead* is disturbing and depressing, but I find it much more entertaining now, perhaps because my memories of those same streets portrayed in the film are no longer reinforced daily. I also feel more sympathy for Frank, Larry, Marcus, and all paramedics sucked into primitive EMS systems that expect employees only to show up and answer calls, with little direction from anyone other than dispirited partners. You have to be at least a little crazy to survive in such an environment.

Skid Marks (2007)

Rating: Not until I grasp the concept of negative stars

Plot summary

Two ambulance companies, "Bayside Ambulatory Life Services" and "Downtown Intensive Care" (BALS and DIC—get it?), are battling over who can transport the most patients, in this infantile caricature of infirmity, ethnicity, and sexuality. The winning agency earns exclusive rights to Bayshore, "Home of America's Greatest Seaman" (yup, I'm still hysterical over that one). Rich, T-Bone, Karl, and One Foot (he's two feet taller than that—I'd explain if I could control my mirth) are the guys with BALS, while Bob and Neil work for DIC.

Sorry, I can't help it. Watching *Skid Marks* makes me think like a 10-year-old, which is a problem because *The Mickey Mouse Club* seems to have gone off the air.

Anyway, the good guys from BALS hang around headquarters and have unprotected sex, while the bad guys from DIC try to stick it to their rivals while having unprotected sex. The difference is that most of the DICs have sex by themselves.

In the name of all that is holy, please make it stop.

Voodoo EMS

This movie could have been *titled* Voodoo EMS. We know it, the actors know it, even the audience knows it (I pray). So let's go the opposite way and highlight a few scenes that are just realistic enough to resemble actual alarms:

- A diff breather in a hospital gown alternates puffs on a cigarette and gulps of O_2.
- One Foot responds to a patient pleasuring himself with a vacuum cleaner. (One of my partners answered a similar alarm, except the hardware of choice was an electric drill. I think the carnage was more traumatic to the crew than the patient.)
- Rich tries tempting a cute co-worker with nebulized vodka. No, I've never seen that, but I'm definitely curious.

Say again?

If you're an EMT with a fragile ego, beware: *Skid Marks* must have been written by a colleague for whom self-loathing is an art form. Here's a sample:

- *"We're EMTs. That's a step, or several stories, below a well-trained paramedic."*—Rich, ruling out any chance of being elected shop steward.
- *"Paramedics [as opposed to EMTs] get paid a salary, have training, and actually save lives."*—Rich to the new guy, who might not have learned as much from that statement as I did.
- *"So I became an EMT, which affords me the luxury of no real responsibility."*—Rich to his eventual girlfriend, who replies, *"You're going to make some lucky girl a great ex-husband."* Point taken.

Subjective assessment

If the measure of a movie is how much it makes you think, *Skid Marks* is a masterpiece. After watching only the first five minutes, I started contemplating the path I had chosen—not the one about becoming a medic; the one about deciding to review this turkey.

By the 15-minute mark, I was thinking up excuses for abandoning the project: the DVD never arrived, my mailbox was stolen, the dog ate my fingers, etc. After 30 minutes, I had to apply pressure to both retinal arteries because my eyes started to bleed. I don't remember much after that.

Skid Marks is a comedy that needs comic relief. Then again, calling such silliness comedy insults all other attempts at humor not dependent on body fluids and bacchanalia. Take whatever money you would have spent on this movie and invest it in Gulf Coast real estate. You'll be better off. And if, like my children, you make a habit of ignoring advice honed by experience, at least wait to watch *Skid Marks* until there's nothing else to try except mowing your lawn with a paring knife.

Mother, Jugs & Speed (1976)

Rating: * * ½

Plot summary

Two ambulance companies are battling over . . . hey, didn't we just see that? No, *Mother, Jugs & Speed* is to *Skid Marks* as champagne is to seltzer. Both are billed as comedies, neither is very funny, but *Mother, Jugs & Speed* captures some very realistic EMS moments, while *Skid Marks* abandons any pretense of accuracy in favor of idiotic gags.

The main characters, Mother, Jugs, and Speed—played by Bill Cosby, Raquel Welch, and Harvey Keitel—work for F&B Ambulance, a mythical Los Angeles EMS agency. For those of you with only second-hand knowledge of the 70s, you'll snicker at the sideburns, disco soundtrack, and leisure suits.

The film tackles gender bias decades before EMS took baby steps in that direction. Jugs endures all the slights and taunts you'd expect someone nicknamed Jugs to suffer. When Harry Fishbine, President of F&B (*Fish* and *Bine*), tells her, "When I get hard-up enough to hire a woman driver, I'll be dead two years," we root for her to change his mind. She does.

Voodoo EMS

By 1976, my only exposure to EMS was when I stopped a hockey puck with my face. I'll have to rely on those of you who learned to sling and swathe while doing The Hustle to tell us whether the following scenes were authentic:

- Two EMTs carry an obese female down several flights of stairs *in a stretcher*—the metal kind with wheels and everything. Just watching that made my back spasm. Had the scoop and stair chair not been invented yet? Even NFL running backs moonlighting as bomb-disposal technicians must have had longer careers than EMTs.
- When an elderly male goes into cardiac arrest en route to the hospital, Speed simply announces, "He's dead," then looks sad. Was thinning the herd a '70s concept I missed?
- I've heard bite sticks were used for seizures back then, but sitting on a patient's legs to control convulsions? Tonic/clonic/moronic, I'd say.

Say again?

Most of the humor in *Mother, Jugs & Speed* is subtle, with side tones of sadness, indignity, frustration, and sociopathy. We get it, and apparently so do the producers. Here's a sample:

- *"That's why I like working for you—because you have no self-respect."*—Mother to Harry, who takes bribes from ambulance-chasing lawyers and pays kickbacks to phony patients, but still gets to work with Raquel Welch every day. So much for karma.
- *"You drive my hours, you listen to my music, and you pay for your own beer."*—Mother to Speed, echoing what every FTO would like to say.
- *"I think you got some trouble down here in your coccyl joint."*—EMT Murdoch to a patient who happens to be a wrestler and female. Even if there were a coccyl joint, I don't think that's what he was touching.

Subjective assessment

I appreciated the realistic scenarios and sporadic, dark humor. Even those of you who are relatively new to EMS will relate to the call-buffing, ER diversion, and hernia-inducing lifting. I commend the cast and crew for doing their homework.

Speaking of the cast, viewers get sneak previews of such rising stars as Larry Hagman, Bruce Davison, and Harvey Keitel. The cameo by ex-linebacker Dick Butkus reminds us that acting isn't as easy as it looks.

Ambulance Girl (2005)

Rating: * * ½

Plot summary

Kathy Bates plays Jane Stern, a bipolar food critic who wants to be a bipolar EMT. While visiting her hometown rescue squad, she meets longtime member Walter, who mollifies Jane's avowed aversion to body fluids by confiding, "Some of us end up heaving our guts out." Stern reluctantly buys into paroxysmal vomiting; joins the Grafton, Connecticut, Volunteer Fire Department; and begins an EMT class. Along the way, she and her husband, fellow foodie Michael, struggle with commitment, resentment, and divergent career paths. EMS is tangential to the film's theme—that self-fulfillment is a by-product of stable relationships.

Voodoo EMS

- Jane treats Michael's hand lac according to the directive, "Do no harm, but if you do, stop doing it as soon as possible." Here's the protocol:

  1. Apply direct pressure.
  2. Cover the wound with all the ice from your freezer.
  3. Elevate the limb, thereby undoing #2.

- In one scene, all the responders in the Grafton ready room are under 30, in shape, and wearing neat, identical uniforms. I've never worked anywhere in EMS where even one of those traits was evident.

- A paramedic concludes his radio report about a conscious trauma patient with, "Blood pressure has not been obtained," just as the camera pans to the IV he's started.

Say again?

- *"You have to be prepared to deal with all sorts of unpleasant sights."*—Walter to Jane, possibly referring to Kathy Bates's nude scene in *About Schmidt*.
- *"BSI, I'm Number One!"*—Gung-ho EMT instructor Ed, exhorting students to echo his inspirational chant. Hey Ed, at least make it rhyme. How about "PPE, I'm in it for me!"?
- *"Scapula, maxilla—I love these words!"*—Jane to an obviously annoyed Michael, who probably thinks she's hinting about male enhancement meds again.

Subjective assessment

Whenever I see Kathy Bates, I think of Annie Wilkes, the deranged nurse who abducts, confines, and cripples James Caan's character in *Misery*. Jane Stern doesn't seem psychotic enough to be played by Ms. Bates. When Ambulance Girl breaks some triage nurse's legs with a sledgehammer, I'll reconsider.

The best actor in this flick is Robin Thomas, who plays Jane's husband. We have a lot in common: His name is Michael and my name is Michael. He's a writer and I'm a writer. He's a great cook . . . and my name is Michael.

I recommend *Ambulance Girl* to conflicted, moderately obsessed, occasionally despondent EMS providers with significant past or current family issues. In other words, most of us.

Daylight (1996)

Rating: * *

Plot summary

Remember Rambo, Sylvester Stallone's commie-crunching, bandolier-brandishing character of the 80s? Did you ever wonder how he would have turned out if, instead of joining the Army's Special Forces and becoming a one-man apocalypse, he'd gone to EMT school? *Daylight* forces us to contemplate that alternative universe.

As former NYC★EMS Chief Kit Latura, Stallone gets to treat, rather than inflict, sucking chest wounds in this disaster flick that will remind people my age of *The Poseidon Adventure*. Instead of an ocean liner, though, the scene is an unnamed Hudson River tunnel looking a lot like the Holland that collapses at both ends after a robbery getaway car collides with a couple of trucks carrying hazmat from Manhattan to Jersey City. Latura, who lost his EMS job after mishandling a South Bronx building collapse, responds Code 3 in his taxi cab to help triage victims at the New York entrance, debates rescue plans with incident commanders, then is asked to lead a mid-shaft rescue after the new EMS boss gets "pancaked" by tunnel debris. And I thought tub/toilet extrications were challenging.

There are obligatory near-death and real-death experiences, tender moments shared by potential soulmates, and soliloquies about life's inequities before this fast-paced film reaches a predictable conclusion. Oh, and there's this really cute dog who sometimes looks like he's eyeing his trapped human companions as dinner.

Voodoo EMS

- Frank, the acting EMS Chief and the guy who had Kit fired, asks Kit if he wants to go into the collapsed tunnel alone, carrying only a few hand tools, to treat survivors and find a way out. It's a Rambo-esque moment when Kit replies, "Give me clearance." I think most of us would have said, "Kiss my trauma shears."

- A soaked, shivering patient pulled from a tunnel escape hatch is given a stat IM injection of . . . what? Hudson River antitoxin?

Say again?

- *"Breaker, breaker, we got a smoker, we got a smoker!"*—George, the cop, to Command. If a fireball the size of a dirigible is "a smoker," then millions of gallons of water engulfing the tunnel must be "a leaker."

- *"You don't achieve what I have without an instinct for torque."*—Roy, a celebrity athlete, to Kit. I don't get this. Maybe he said, "an instinct for *pork*." In any case, Roy's instincts weren't that good, considering he's a mountain climber who couldn't even find his way to sea level.

• *"Hey Mikey, you think we're pretty?"*—It doesn't matter who said it; I just like the sound of it.

Subjective assessment

You know what you're going to get from Stallone, and it ain't Shakespeare in the Park ("Yo, Lord—what fools these mortals be, absolutely!"). He doesn't disappoint when the script calls for super-human stunts or even strenuous grunting, but dialogue still isn't his strength.

Daylight got an Oscar nomination for Best Sound Effects Editing. Also for Best Retriever in a Non-Speaking Role.

Author's Note

In my review of Skid Marks, you'll notice a snide remark about investing in Gulf Coast real estate. That was in 2010, soon after the Deepwater Horizon disaster. I'd just lost a few thousand bucks on BP stock and wasn't in a charitable mood.

Mother, Jugs & Speed is the film I felt closest to due to its familiar portrayal of the 70s, when I had four respectable jobs, a Captain and Tennille eight-track, and a yellow leisure suit for dancing the night away and getting down with my bad self, or something like that.

DECONSTRUCTING HEROISM

2016

D id you see this headline a few months ago?

Honeymoon Hero: Bride responds to crash

The story is about a Tennessee medic who stopped at a wreck on the way from her wedding. The patient turned out to be a family member who suffered "major bumps and bruises."

The bride says she's not a hero. I believe her. It's not the "bumps and bruises" part that disqualifies her; it's the danger to the rescuer, or lack of it. To be a hero, I think you have to face an outcome more onerous than a smudged wedding dress.

To me, heroism is a demonstrated willingness to risk one's life for another. That doesn't happen very often in EMS, yet our field is overstocked with novice responders who equate EMS with lifesaving, and lifesaving with heroism. I bet those unmet expectations hasten early retirement as much as bad backs and low pay.

Nonchalant anointing of heroes didn't start with EMS; it's part of a nationwide trend toward sensationalism rooted in news and entertainment media's competition for your attention. As a result, our society often equates admirable behavior with valor worthy of kisses on both cheeks. *Hero*, once a meaningful term that evoked images of selfless sacrifice, has been overused to the point of having no more significance than *great* or *super*. If Clark Kent could even find a phone booth today, he'd have to emerge as *Totally* Superman just to compete with all the other "super" men and women.

Calling someone a hero on the six o'clock news is mostly an excuse for a provocative sound bite. I wish I were immune to such tactics, but I'm just as likely as anyone to look up from my smartphone when I hear the H word on TV. Suddenly I'm wondering who did what for whom. Game point to the talking head with the teaser.

Even if you've behaved heroically at least once, you probably don't wake up every morning yearning to duplicate that feat. There must be something besides bravery keeping you in uniform. Could we distill your positive energy—your willingness to do this job without applause—into hypothetical sound bites for our own people? Let's try.

EMT Still Polite After 20 Years

Ralph K of ABC Ambulance routinely greets patients warmly and asks what he can do for them.

> *"Most are good people," the EMT says. "They don't know much about EMS; they just need some help. You shouldn't be in this job if you don't want to help."*

Paramedic Takes Classes Not Required

An Adams County paramedic confirms she signed up for sociology and psychology courses not because she had to, but because she wants to understand people better.

> *"There's lots of stuff we learn in medic school, but it never seems to be enough," says Susie C. "I just figured it was time to get into more of the science—what makes people tick, what they need, why they do what they do. Maybe that'll help me take care of them."*

Dispatcher Puts Callers at Ease

When Frank M answers East Ogden's 9-1-1 line, he uses cue cards to determine the nature of each emergency. But callers don't know they're supposed to follow a script.

"Last night I took a call from an elderly woman with chest pain who asked if I knew when the next train from the city was due," Frank says. "Her son was supposed to be on it. I found a website with the timetable and was able to answer her question. It was no big deal."

Ambulance Boss Gives Employees "Mental Health" Days

Robin T knows what it's like to need a break from EMS.

"I rode for 20 years before starting this company," the owner of ABC Ambulance says. "Sometimes you just have to get away, even for a day. I'm pretty understanding about sick time when employees work extra shifts to help out."

The world is so desperately short of real heroes, we accept all kinds of pseudo-courageous behavior as substitutes for the real thing. Sometimes EMS providers get caught in the middle—between heroic and dependable—because we're an industry in search of a label, and *America's Finest* is already taken.

We can give our rare, true heroes their deserved honors without overlooking the steady, compassionate competence of those who care for others every shift. More than heroism, that's what everyone watching the six o'clock news will need someday.

INFORMED DISSENT

2014

I have a case I'd like to discuss with you. Except for a few members of the patient's family, you'll be the first to hear about it. I'm going to withhold certain details that might reveal the patient's identity.

The 57-year-old female—we'll call her Helen—had complained of intermittent, severe, lower abdominal pain for several weeks. She was diagnosed with perforation of a very important organ—less important than her stomach, more important than her gall bladder—and was admitted to a hospital in the capital city of a mid-southern state known for its music. I won't say what kind of major surgery Helen had; you'll find a clue in this sentence.

Not only is my wife a good sport, she's also a former EMT and EMD who's not shy about critiquing healthcare—particularly her own. Helen agreed to let me trash her confidentiality so we could discuss how some of her in-patient experiences relate to prehospital practices.

Until the day of her operation, Helen was treated well by the medical-industrial complex. It wasn't until she entered the hospital that The System, aware Helen now bore the mark of the infirm around her wrist, took steps to subordinate her by exploiting patients' lowest common denominator: neediness. The more help she needed, the longer it took to get help. I'm not sure why; I can only speculate some of her caregivers saw their work as inherently confrontational. By enforcing pointlessly inflexible policy, they asserted control.

Want to speak with your attending physician—the one on a first-name basis with your intestines? Don't call direct. If you do, your doctor's receptionist will transfer you back to a floor nurse to take a message for—you guessed it—your attending physician.

Due for another shot of morphine in five minutes? Don't even think about pressing the call button yet. I'd have more respect for such contrived precision if my wife wasn't routinely kept waiting 20 minutes or more after her meds were due.

I've seen EMS providers' rote adherence to procedures degenerate into us-against-them clashes with patients prehospitally, too. I might have fostered some of those negative vibes when I thought I was merely enforcing treatment or transport policies. For example, am I favoring safety or convenience if I automatically discourage bathroom breaks for patients before transport, or bar family from bench seats? The easier it becomes to say no, the harder it is to remember why.

Most of the inpatient absurdities Helen endured were more annoying than dangerous, but some were scary. A few hours after waking up in recovery, Helen noticed part of her left thigh was numb. Her doctor said not to worry, then resumed rounds. A few days later, Helen suddenly developed edema in that leg. Her nurse said not to worry while giving report to the next shift.

I didn't know the etiology of Helen's complications, but I probably wasn't going to be convinced by anyone that numbness and edema so far from a surgical site met popular criteria for normal. What Helen and I needed was someone with advanced medical training to focus on her long enough to at least give us the impression her complaints were understood and would be addressed.

Lack of focus can be a problem prehospitally, too. Most of us have been seduced by calls that sound more interesting than the ones we're on. Sometimes we have to remind ourselves that victims of "routine" illness or injury probably won't appreciate whatever shortcuts we think we're taking for the greater good.

Is it possible to spend enough time with every patient? Probably not, but I can't see setting an arbitrary limit of, say, 15 minutes, as the sign at one doctor's office stated. Surely, face time should be dictated by something other than a ticking clock.

I realize fiscal realities intrude on almost all good intentions. However, after watching Helen struggle to be recognized as an individual, rather than as a transaction, I'm thinking medicine wasn't meant to be a business. Sometimes it seems too difficult to care for people properly *and* profitably. Early physician-theologians had it right when they offered primitive healthcare as charitable acts instead of provider-centric indulgences. Wellness lags behind technology when patients are merely processed.

Like you, I have a whole new year to get a better handle on this.

Author's Note

Regarding that clue about Helen's surgery at the end of the second paragraph, some of you swear it's not there. You mean you didn't notice the semicolon?

I wish I could say we've had better experiences with caregivers during the past seven years, but there have been too many misunderstandings to make Helen and I feel anything other than dread when we're at the mercy of medical professionals. The older we get, the more vulnerable we seem to be.

GOODNESS AND LIGHT

2014

Last May, my good friend Cliff became a grandfather for the second time. He describes the experience as "joy without the fear" new parents feel. As an *old* parent, I'm intrigued. As an old *paramedic*, I don't think I'll ever be as comfortable with grandchildren as Cliff. The stakes still seem pretty high to me when I'm taking care of someone else's child.

I bring this up because as Christmas approaches, I think of kids—not snow or reindeer or maxed-out credit cards. Children, especially little ones enjoying another year of magical thinking, take to Christmas like tadpoles to water.

My daughter's uncompromised delight at the holidays always made me smile. Her health and happiness were the best gifts I ever got. I figured Christmas was my reward for 364 other days of problem-solving and sacrifice that are part of every parent's job description.

Working over Christmas was a consequence of choosing EMS over more family-friendly occupations. I'd approach holiday duty like other shifts, hoping not to screw up, then add a holiday wish for no pediatric patients. Tragedies involving children were hard enough to process without linkage to annual events. I didn't need any help remembering my worst kid calls.

In 1993, just months after joining EMS, I treated a 12-year-old pedestrian struck by a car. I had to bag him all the way to the hospital because he was paralyzed from the neck down. My daughter was only a year younger; perhaps that's why my clinical detachment was overwhelmed by paternal concern. I visited him in the hospital every day until a senior coworker told me I'd have too many patients to care that much about each one. I thought to myself, *Fine, only the kids then.*

Two years later, I was nearing the end of medic school when I was assigned to a peds floor during hospital rotations. There was this little guy who had suffered a stroke before his first birthday. He was two years old with not much more than a sucking reflex to indicate responsiveness. One day, he stopped breathing during a CT scan, then brady-ed down just as we'd been taught children would. The nurse standing with me was less prepared than I was to actually use some of the PALS I'd just studied.

Then there was the 15-year-old girl in 2003 who couldn't think of a reason to live past November. She climbed through a bedroom window onto the roof of her house and hung herself from a backyard tree. A small, stuffed bear dangled from a branch next to hers—an obvious plea for help found too late to make a difference. That was Helen's last call.

My scariest kid case actually ended well. I was transporting a sick one-year-old with his parents. The mother, who'd been holding the child during transport (the custom in those days), handed me her son at the hospital so she could safely exit our ambulance. When she had trouble with the big step in back, I stupidly sat the baby on the rear-facing captain's chair so I could assist mom.

As I walked from the front of the cabin to the double doors in back, my fidgety patient fell from his seat with an audible thud. The child wasn't hurt, but his screams so terrorized and angered his parents, they laid into me as if I were Darth Vader channeling Hannibal Lecter. I started to imagine round after round of discipline beginning at my agency and ending at Sing Sing. I was lucky the only consequence of my carelessness was a well-deserved apology to the parents.

My wife and I still celebrate Christmas, but in my opinion, it's a holiday for children. Innocent and uninhibited, young ones don't suspect bad intent of strangers bearing gifts. Kids know joy grown-ups can't remember. I think most adults are suspicious of good fortune; we can't help second-guessing ourselves even when life is good. It's as if we cash in our cheerfulness chips to pay for passage from youth.

As I drive around town, I see a familiar Christmas landscape: city streets sprouting evergreen canopies as suburban homeowners compete for most colorful use of kilowatts. I have many good memories of colleagues, family, and friends, but my Dickensian regard for Christmas Past still centers on Tiny Tim's plight.

Merry Christmas to sons and daughters everywhere. Merry Christmas to parents and grandparents who care.

Author's Note

In 2016, Helen and I became grandparents for the first time. Cliff was right: It's fun and not hard. Grandkids are easy to love; plus, they go home at night. It's a wonderful arrangement— one that we're enjoying twice as much after the birth of grandson number two.

PAST
IMPERFECT

2010

A third of the way through medic school, I had to show I could handle a simulated megacode—a cardiac arrest that morphs from one lethal arrhythmia to another. My instructor sat patiently as I verbalized every bit of personal protection not requiring a carry permit, performed a quick look on a chronically unresponsive manikin, defibrillated a disorganized rhythm I prayed wasn't pulseless electrical artifact, delegated CPR to imaginary probies, started an IV on a disembodied arm, then pushed a milligram of epinephrine because ineffectiveness wasn't a contraindication.

"Mike," my examiner said as I considered my next lifesaving intervention, "do you know what a mulligan is?"

A drug? A fish? I had no idea.

"Not a golfer, eh? A mulligan's a second chance, and you just got one. Don't waste it."

In a nanosecond, I realized I'd committed the most egregious of scenario-based sins: failure to control the airway. I should have oxygenated and intubated my synthetic patient immediately after directing my phantom crew to start chest compressions. With my preceptor's permission, I backed up a bit and demonstrated my ability to ventilate through the correct hole.

Today, I'm wishing I'd had a few more mulligans, because that omission—serious enough 16 years ago to almost cost me a passing grade—is now standard of care. It says so in the American Heart Association's 2005 version of Advanced Cardiac Life Support. Not only do we delay invasive airway management, but also pulse checks, rhythm reinterpretation, medication administration, and patient movement, so chest compressions aren't interrupted for more than 10 seconds at a time. I don't know how many cardiac arrests I ran before 2005—a hundred, perhaps—but I'm quite sure we stopped CPR for much longer than 10 seconds at least once during every one of them.

Soon we'll be introduced to another iteration of ACLS. It happens every five years—longer than the average bear market, shorter than the life cycle of North American cicadas. Is there a reason, other than reliance on a decimal system, that we commit to new algorithms for half a decade per revision? Would we be saving more lives if our founding fathers had favored three-dollar bills or counted to four instead of ten when they were angry?

Another major change in cardiac arrest management has been reduction in the ratio of breaths to compressions. In 2005, I learned, like many of you, that we'd been bagging our patients too aggressively and inhibiting venous return by building intrathoracic pressure. That's good to know. I would have stopped squeezing the bag so vigorously a year earlier had my protocols echoed research published in 2004.

Having helped author prehospital policies, I realize changing a region's scope of practice requires years of lead time for study, debate, and training. There must be a way, though, to institute top-down, emergent "recalls" of questionable advice whenever a new consensus emerges. As EMTs and paramedics, we're not permitted to make those decisions ourselves. If we were, I guarantee you a bunch of us would have stopped administering meds endotracheally long before the '05 version of ACLS labeled that route much less effective than IV or IO.

Maybe there's a solution close to home. Have you noticed your computer downloading software patches automatically, often before those bugs affect you? Couldn't we also treat protocols dynamically, relying more on real-time updates than periodic hard-copy revisions? An email announcing version 12.34 of standing orders wouldn't be a bad way to highlight changes not requiring supplementary skills or training.

I'm wondering what therapeutic interventions will be added and which tenets of acute care will be discredited by the AHA this year. How wrong have we been since 2005? Since 2000? For example, will ACLS encourage use of passive ventilation instead of positive pressure during some cardiac arrests? I hope so, because new research shows the odds of survival among patients who present in ventricular fibrillation are greater if we stow the BVM and start with a non-rebreather. That would have been considered ridiculous and possibly career threatening when I joined EMS. Now, passive ventilation looks like the way to begin fresh arrests, but we'll probably have to wait another year or two for regional standards to conform. Is there anything individual EMS providers can do to expedite that process?

Yes. Stay close to the literature between ACLS rewrites. Be opportunistic about questioning local practices that haven't quite caught up to cutting-edge medicine. Find sympathetic physicians with regulatory or advisory responsibilities, then play what-if with them to explore innovative discretionary orders short term, followed by provisional protocol updates. If those of us in the field don't show initiative, who will?

The 2010 version of ACLS might be my last as a medic according to my tormentors, L5 and S1. Even if I forget an algorithm or two, I'll try to remember what Austrian philosopher Karl Raimund Popper said about making mistakes, a few years before EMS was invented: "Science is one of the very few human activities . . . in which errors are systematically criticized and fairly often, in time, corrected."

Until we run out of second chances.

Author's Note

By the time I'd been through four more updates, I felt ACLS (and PALS) had become reservoirs of questionable practices and wishful thinking. A bigger problem was the one-size-fits-all philosophy that placed me in a class with 10 nurses. Imagine truckers reviewing rules of the road with motorcyclists.

Some instructors seemed to be stuck in time warps, with less mastery of current practices than memories of discredited ones. It was up to students—skeptical paramedic-journalists, especially—to point out discrepancies between tired lectures and current thinking.

The next two chapters describe my most recent alphabet-course updates. They were funny at times, but never fun.

ACLS 2018
DID YOU HEAR THE ONE ABOUT THE MEDIC AND THE ABG?

2018

Whenever it's time to refresh my ACLS credentials, I get all nostalgic. Mostly, I remember those megacodes from paramedic school 24 years ago, when evil instructors used diabolical rhythm generators to assault helpless manikins. Even worse, we students were complicit. We hastened the demise of Rescue Annie and her anatomically ambiguous friends by inflicting intubation, stacked shocks, lidocaine, bretylium, sodium bicarbonate, and other pseudo-scientific therapies on lifeless and legless torsos, while calling for chest compressions only when convenient.

Fast forward to 2018, and *bretylium* isn't even a word anymore, according to my dictionary. Bicarb amps sit unused at the bottom of drug bags until they break or expire. Those are just two examples of how much cardiac arrest protocols have changed since the '90s. Today, we believe long-term survival mostly depends on uninterrupted CPR and prompt defibrillation. Intubation? Only if you have time. Ventilation? All you need is a BVM. Medications?

Medications? Anyone?

That's what irks me most about my 2018 ACLS update. There's still no evidence epinephrine or antiarrhythmics offer pulseless patients anything more than slightly slower death, yet those drugs remain at the core of AHA cardiac arrest algorithms. Why? Is there nothing more useful we could be offering impressionable clinicians during 16 hours of minimally invasive learning? How about some practice with supraglottic airways or an IV clinic focusing on meds for the living? And shouldn't we be hearing something about ECMO?

I could write a much longer article than this one about the frailty of ACLS; how we spent decades doing resuscitation wrong and are still wasting our time with therapeutics short on evidence. That wouldn't be news to most of you, though, so here's your headline: There's nothing new in ACLS 2018, other than a couple of re-engineered videos starring computer-generated avatars as brave paramedics. Yes, these are exciting times for androids.

It's easy to find humor in ACLS if you don't get too bogged down by science. We're talking about a course that tries to teach one set of stilted algorithms and rote responses to doctors, paramedics, nurses, PAs, respiratory therapists, dentists, pharmacists, athletic trainers, and anyone else who can memorize 15-20 unambiguous EKGs in time for the pretest. It's absurd to have a common curriculum for every kind of healthcare professional. Try spending a couple of days playing "manikin down" with caregivers who've never run a real arrest, and the jokes will write themselves.

I'll Take Blood Work for $200, Alex

The AHA wants us to consider "H's and T's"—10 presumptive diagnoses beginning with those letters—whenever we have nothing else to do during hopelessly contrived scenarios, which is often. I get the part about mulling etiologies, but when I mentioned pulmonary emboli as one cause of PEA, that didn't mean I knew which labs to order. ABG? CBC? MTV? You have to go to a different school for that. Here's a clue for my fellow street medics: D-dimer is a blood test, not a rapper.

Hurry Up and Wait

The most frustrating part about practicing the AHA's special brand of bogus megacodes is the artificial regimentation that enforces two minutes of CPR (timed by the preceptor) and little else between shocks. You're allowed to start an IV/IO or push one med—but not both—during each interval. And don't even think about intubating unless your imaginary partner is having imaginary problems with the BVM.

After verbalizing the one intervention you're permitted per defibrillation attempt, there's not much else to do, so you get silly. At least I did. I'd tell my five-member team—you know, just like the one on the ambulance—to draw up adenosine and atropine in case my polyurethane patient woke up with either bradycardia or SVT—two rhythms we were told to expect. It definitely helped to know the outcomes in advance.

Everyone Gets a Save

Speaking of survival, my instructor displayed exceptional optimism: Every megacode ended with ROSC. You might think you're home free when you're told there's a pulse, but not so fast; you must verbalize *targeted temperature management.* That's the new name for therapeutic hypothermia, which we now know is not so therapeutic prehospitally. And don't forget to call for "an expert consult." In the field, you and your partner would have to decide which one's the expert.

Advice for Those with Plenty of Liability Insurance

Some of the most entertaining moments in ACLS are when hospital-based educators go off-script to share unique insights. For example, while reviewing signs and symptoms of unstable tachycardia, our teacher told us "a little bit of chest pain is okay." That's probably based on the theory that coronary perfusion is overrated. My favorite tidbit, though, was how third-degree heart block is like "two people getting divorced." Trust me, it's not that simple.

It's healthy to laugh at ACLS while you're still playing paramedic. Here's why: Someday, after you've answered all the calls and carried all the patients your body can take, you're going to tally the pros and cons of your career. You'll remember how good it felt running your first code, but you'll wish someone who'd skipped ACLS had been there to warn you, "That's not how this works; that's not how any of this works."

PALS 2018
HOOKED ON MNEMONICS

2018

Ah, PALS. Like a couple of old friends, we get together every two years and swap stories: You tell me how pediatric assessment is about algorithms and acronyms, and I tell anyone who'll listen that it doesn't work that way. I guess I'm not much of a friend after all.

I just finished my 2018 refresher at a local hospital. My fellow students were mostly nurses, but I didn't mind. I liked being the class's pet paramedic. It was heartwarming to watch my stock rise from creepy old guy to ambulance driver to EMT to "How do you remember all this stuff?" Besides, after decades of being force-fed prehospital war stories by cranky chiefs, it's invigorating to hear about messy ostomies and malfunctioning Foleys from dedicated RNs. Such interdisciplinary bonding is my favorite part of PALS—a course that wants to be practical but, in my opinion, is much more of an intellectual exercise.

In case you missed the memo, the American Heart Association is replacing its five-year cycles of ACLS and PALS revisions with continuous online updates. The good news is, there haven't been any significant changes to PALS since 2015. That's also the bad news because PALS 2018 presents with familiar weaknesses:

> **One course for all caregivers.** PALS should have separate tracks for hospital and prehospital personnel. Nurses hardly ever intubate or run arrests, and most medics don't order lab work, give antibiotics, or monitor patients beyond admission.

> **A contrived focus on sequence of care.** This is a problem with EMS training, too. Students are taught mnemonics and acronyms as if patient care necessarily follows sequential patterns. In PALS, it's *EII (Evaluate, Identify, Intervene)*, *CAB* with

a side order of *H's* and *T's, ABCDE, AVPU,* and *SAMPLE.* During practice scenarios, instructors wanted to hear what letter we were on, not how we'd use our bedside spidey sense to drive assessment. SMH.

Not enough props for practical exercises. It's hard enough to do PALS without real patients. Subtract realistic manikins, monitors, and supplies—missing or malfunctioning in every AHA class I've attended—and someone needs to ask what the point is. I vote for reimagining the course as a moderated seminar, where students sit in a circle, review algorithms, discuss recent developments in their little corners of the medical-industrial complex, and play a few rounds of Name That Disease.

Therapy with little or no proven value. When I first took PALS in 1994, we were taught to give kids in cardiac arrest epinephrine—sometimes in massive doses. Here's what the AHA warns about that drug 24 years later: "No adult or pediatric studies have demonstrated improved survival (after cardiac arrest) with use of epinephrine." The same could be said about lidocaine and amiodarone, yet you can fail PALS if you don't verbalize prompt administration of all three meds.

Despite our class's professional bearing and reverence for all anatomically correct life forms, there were some amusing moments:

- We were watching a video about the value of teamwork (also the value of having four nurses and a physician gowned up and waiting in the ED for an incoming cardiac arrest). As the EMS crew arrived with CPR in progress and prepared to slide their patient from the stretcher to the hospital gurney, the MD who was playing the stoic team leader told them, "Let's wait until you get to 30 [compressions]." That doc should do a few ride-alongs. Even the actors portraying EMTs looked like they were thinking, *Seriously?*
- I've heard EKGs described by novice caregivers as "camel humps," "little fire hats," and now, for the second time from a PALS instructor, "goats holding hands" (v-tach, of course).

How precious. What's next, "The Cat in the Hat Does an Amiodarone Drip"?

- As we were practicing megacodes, our monitor suddenly sounded an alarm and displayed the message, *Shutting down now*. Then there was a burning smell. We couldn't recall any defibrillator-on-fire memory aids, so we improvised RA for *run away*.
- Being a saver of lives, I was ordered to demonstrate endotracheal intubation on a decapitated polyurethane patient. I was struggling to visualize the cords—difficult on a free-floating head—when my instructor suggested I stop "trying to do it the right way" and just lean the blade against the teeth.

After my biennial bolus of PALS, I'm still not comfortable with incisors as fulcrums, but when the tones go out for "manikin down," I'm your huckleberry.

Author's Note

My ACLS and PALS refreshers were only a month apart—not enough time for rehab. Please excuse my unrelenting cynicism and somewhat repetitive theme.

SHOWING UP

2009

Rob is a paramedic in middle Tennessee, not far from where I live. Some folks kid him about his New York accent. Rob doesn't mind; at most, he'll remind his southern friends why Jefferson Davis's portrait isn't on any U.S. currency.

On the second Tuesday of September, Rob will answer alarms as he did eight years ago, but this time there won't be any 110-story buildings falling on his head. As happy as that makes Rob, his mother is even more relieved. She knows that the invincibility of youth is vulnerable to maladies and madmen.

Rob was one of the most seriously injured 9/11 responders transported to hospitals east of New York City. I know because I was the county administrator assigned to keep track of those things. As Long Island's command-and-control apparatus geared up for an influx of casualties, terse updates from area hospitals lead to a grim conclusion: No one was dying because no one had lived.

When the second of two jetliners struck the Twin Towers, I received a frantic voicemail from my home district's EMS agency to get my gluteus maximus on an ambulance bound for Manhattan. I couldn't comply because I was running medical control 50 miles to the east. It bothered me, though, to be managing my little corner of the crisis from a desk, rather than in the field. My role as a medic, hard-wired to my psyche since Day One of didactics, was rescue.

I picture EMS personnel sizing up Ground Zero, their hands-on bias rendered impotent by medical and environmental factors beyond their control. They encountered the ultimate uncontrolled scene. Their perseverance was remarkable, yet I'm not sure those rescuers ever got enough credit for meeting two of our profession's basic criteria:

> **They showed up.** Woody Allen once attributed 80% of success to showing up. His point, I think, was that successful outcomes involve risk. How many people fleeing lower Manhattan on 9/11 embraced uncertainty and reversed course to help others?

> **They adapted.** We tell the uninitiated that EMS isn't for everyone because of graphic trauma and devastating illness, but the chaos quotient is an obstacle, too. Exceptional EMS providers prepare to be surprised, deceived, enticed, endangered, alarmed, and appalled. They understand that adapting to the unexpected is a full-time job.

Before I got started in EMS, I was a card-carrying member of corporate America. For us, adapting meant getting accustomed to a new office, a different boss, or heart-healthy cuisine in the cafeteria. There were inconveniences and indignities, but nothing like you might find at an MCI. Achieving competence in an industrial environment isn't complicated; it's mostly about learning lines, like a character in a long-running play.

If the business world is Broadway, EMS would be a night at the Improv—no script, only guidelines buttressed by the players' talents and instincts. Our roles are dynamic: students one day and teachers the next; drivers one shift and technicians the next; hand-holders one call and lifesavers the next. Perhaps our toughest task is staying ready, waiting for someone or something to prompt our next move.

EMS has its charm. The after-action high can be exhilarating, the camaraderie is compelling, the tools are cool, and the pay is . . . did I mention the camaraderie? If it were possible to live that life without having to mortgage one's mental and physical well-being, everyone would do it. But responding to emergencies is an unnatural act. The fact that we pay people for that—to show up even when disaster threatens their own families—does not diminish their contributions.

I've participated in dozens of drills designed to simulate death and destruction. I doubt that any amount of moulage can prepare one for an apocalyptic scenario. I don't know of an EMS curriculum that includes "Introduction to Skyscraper Collapse" or "Ballistic

Airliners 101." WTC responders confronted casualties and risks well beyond the scope of their job descriptions; yet they embraced unfamiliar roles as our nation's first agents of homeland security, armed only with expectations of survival. We remember them with admiration and compassion.

Rob, our transplanted medic, isn't only a survivor; he's my son. He showed up, adapted, and played his role. That makes me very proud.

Author's Note

This was the first of several columns I wrote about 9/11 from the 10th anniversary through the 15th. You'll find the others inserted at appropriate intervals.

TALKING BACK

2013

As I write this, I'm six weeks into my annual holiday bout with sciatica. I'm not sure why my Christmases have become so emphatically un-jolly. All I know is my new favorite stocking stuffer is Vicodin.

I mention my less-than-robust state because I know many of you suffer from similar or worse work-related maladies. I'm trying to find the humor in mine.

Here's what I've learned about having a bad back:

- The Borg scale should go to 11.
- Dogs understand your yelping.
- Children lift things you can't.
- Easy chairs are anything but.
- You bend over to pick something up and wonder what else you should do while you're down there (thanks to country legend Little Jimmy Dickens for that one).

I have an L5/S1 herniation that irritates my left sciatic nerve. Usually, there's just mild, intermittent discomfort, but when it flares up, I seriously consider felonious acts against the partners who taught me to use stair chairs instead of stretchers to load patients onto ambulances. Then I embark on a routine of pills in the morning, pills at night, and a cane by my side, all of which can become crutches.

Being away from EMS is almost as frustrating as not being able to do simple chores around the house. The last time I was recovering from sciatica, The Lovely Helen asked me to drag an old, gas grill to the curb. I said that sounded like a good way to pay down the year's health insurance deductible. She thought that was pretty funny. Then she got a neighbor to move it—a middle-aged, petite female neighbor. My ego took a direct hit. I told Helen I'd probably need little blue pills for life. She offered to buy them.

(Memo to significant others: It's risky to make fun of gimpy paramedics. We're sensitive, and we carry needles.)

This year was different because I ended up horizontal in an ambulance just before Thanksgiving. It was an act of desperation; my usual right-lateral-recumbent contortions to curb pain had no effect, and I couldn't sit or stand long enough for Helen to drive me to my doctor.

I was extremely reluctant to call 9-1-1. I suppose that had something to do with all the abuses we see. Also, the thought of entering the system—the same system I'd been a part of for so long—made me feel self-conscious and vulnerable. I didn't want to be someone else's patient.

After promising Helen not to micromanage my own care, I asked her to use the non-emergency number of the dispatch office where she'd worked. Then I considered slipping into something less comfortable but more fashionable for transport, before yielding to the notion of underwear as outerwear.

Here's how I'd grade the performance of my community's medical services:

EMS: *A–.* Courteous, gentle, no mindless back-boarding, and they took me to the hospital of my choice. The only problem was they didn't have any good drugs. Or maybe they did, but I didn't qualify. I knew I shouldn't have offered to slide from my bed to the stretcher.

ED admission: *B.* No waiting for a bay, triaged on the way, and my nurse agreed a rectal exam wouldn't be good for either of us. I was starting to hate hospitals less when someone from billing badgered me about a down payment after my wife had presented our insurance.

Treatment: *A.* The attending physician ordered morphine and steroids right away—even before the x-ray—and two nurses made sure I got my meds promptly. The shots didn't help much, but I appreciated the sense of urgency.

Discharge: *Something at the end of the alphabet.* While Helen went to fetch clothing more substantial than underwear for my trip home, I was banished to the waiting room to . . . uh . . . wait. If you'd been there, you would have seen this scary-looking, barefoot guy in a t-shirt and paper pants—the best the hospital could offer to preserve my modesty. I tried not to look like an extra from *One Flew Over the Cuckoo's Nest*, but I did notice mothers shielding their children.

Today is special: It's my first day back at work in over a month. I was supposed to wait another week, but some of our people are in worse shape than I am. No problem, I'm ready. I'm eager to engage. I want to show everyone I can do all the things I did before.
Or maybe I'll just try standing up straight.

Author's Note
My return to work was brief; I resigned less than a month later due to ongoing back trouble.

THE 800-HOUR EMT

2016

Breakfast is my favorite time because it's the first chance The Lovely Helen and I have each day to discuss matters of interest. We take turns making the coffee: I do it when she's in Kazakhstan and she does it all the other times.

This morning's topic was EMS, which only gets mentioned on days starting with capital letters. Usually we talk about calls we shared and people we knew, but just to be different, I floated an idea so compelling, Helen could only conclude, "You must have had help—you're not that clever."

I'd suggested to Helen that we eliminate what has become an artificial distinction between ALS and BLS, and have only one class of personnel on 9-1-1 ambulances in most of the U.S. I'm not the first to suggest that, but I might be the oldest. Feel free to humor me as you would your great-uncle who keeps telling you to buy sensible shoes.

My retooled EMS provider—closer to paramedic than EMT—would get approximately 800 hours of instruction compared to the 1,000-1,400 hours offered today. That's the opposite of the direction favored by most deep thinkers I know.

Why take a giant step backwards in training? Because I think we've pretty much maxed out the responsibilities we can give medical practitioners without higher education, and I don't see a consensus on degree requirements anytime soon. After two decades, at least, of artificially inflating paramedics' responsibilities with superficial instruction in difficult-to-master skills for rarely encountered conditions, I believe it's time to focus on a smaller subset of presenting problems.

Before you start sending me strident email, let me explain that last sentence.

Artificially inflating the role of paramedics. I mean a curriculum that makes "basic" paramedics with 9-1-1 tool sets seem more skilled than we are. Should I have standing orders for atropine when mildly symptomatic patients present with heart rates in the 40s? No. How about amiodarone drips for tachycardic patients not sick enough for cardioversion? Probably not.

Superficial instruction. The average U.S. paramedic program doesn't have enough hours or equipment to rigorously cover all therapeutics within the syllabus. Teachers aren't to blame; most do the best they can with the tools and time they're given, but some high-risk procedures and seldom seen conditions within paramedics' scope of practice are barely mentioned.

What would we delete from the current curriculum? The most demanding care for unlikely prehospital ailments; meconium aspiration, for example. Most paramedics don't have enough experience with neonates to reliably intubate and suction them.

Let's get rid of cricothyrotomies, too—needle and surgical. How much practice do most of us get in that? One could even argue *all* prehospital advanced airway management should be restricted to inserting supraglottic devices, but we'd better wait for further research on carotid-artery impairment by SGDs.

I'd also discontinue prehospital treatment of unstable arrhythmias with anything but electricity, and eliminate IV infusions of any kind. EKG interpretations would focus on immediate threats to life.

I was going to suggest 700 hours of training instead of 800, but I'd want to leave room for enhanced behavioral and well-care topics like psychology, sociology, public health, and even communication. What could be more important than learning how to relate to the people we're treating?

Lowering, rather than raising, prehospital standards of care would almost certainly position EMS as a trade rather than a profession. That would be a relief to colleagues not seeking higher education. Bachelor's degrees would continue to be the gateway for those wishing to practice at more advanced levels, like nurses, physician assistants, or MDs. Speaking of RNs, they'd not only staff high-risk transports, but run them.

Think of the operational simplicity: No ALS or BLS buses. Anyone who calls an ambulance gets the same level of care. Partners have equal opportunities for practice. No decisions about ALS intercepts. No more arguments about what skills belong under which certification level. And as a bonus, no more slogans about EMTs saving paragods.

The transition from current EMR–EMT-AEMT-paramedic classifications would be straightforward: Paramedics would devote their next refreshers to the hundred-or-so hours of socially responsible coursework mentioned above; all others would have to upgrade or do something else for a living. This might be a good time to buy stock in companies selling bridge courses.

EMS agencies would establish the market for the new class of prehospital worker. Salaries would fall between those of today's EMTs and paramedics.

Let's teach all our prehospital providers to master the same realistic subset of prehospital care and embrace the nobility of EMS as an essential *trade*.

Okay, now you can send me that email.

Author's Note

That's exactly what happened. Although there was constructive feedback from some readers about how my plan could be improved for rural areas, I got more hate mail than anyone not responsible for raising taxes.

The next column provoked a similar reaction.

STUCK IN REVERSE

2016

I think I may have gotten EMS backwards.

For a long time, I assumed volunteers were contributing to lower wages in our industry by increasing the supply of EMS workers relative to demand. I even conceded that the number of paid paramedic and EMT positions are limited by willingness of volunteers to do our jobs for nothing.

What if the reverse were true? What if paid EMS providers were encroaching on a service that's meant to be all volunteer?

Before you start wondering if I'm a victim of long-term Nitronox exposure, return with me—conceptually, at least—to a simpler time, when prehospital care for emergent patients was little more than oxygen and a stretcher. I'm thinking of the 1950s, when there really were ambulance drivers, but no EMTs, paramedics, or other physician extenders because it was widely assumed any training short of medical school was insufficient to diagnose and treat most illnesses and injuries.

One thing I remember about those days is my mother taking an American Red Cross first-aid course, the precursor of today's EMT curriculum. She wasn't thinking of becoming a professional "first-aider"; there was no such thing. She just wanted to be able to help, as a concerned citizen, if she witnessed a medical emergency. I know that because she said so while she practiced her sling-and-swathe on me.

I don't remember Mom ever using her first-aid skills, but there were plenty of times she brought my brothers and me to the doctor's office. She must have understood first-aid involved mostly superficial steps not meant to substitute for physicians' definitive care. If she'd thought nascent prehospital services were more therapeutic than what she'd learned to do, she would have summoned ambulances on several occasions when my brothers and I found novel ways to bleed. She never did.

The advent of EMS in the late 60s broadened the concept of citizen first-aid to include state-certified specialists with 80 hours or more of emergency medical training. By the time paramedics were appearing in the early 70s, the public's expectations of prehospital interventions were beginning to exceed stopgap measures and were approaching definitive care for some cardiac, respiratory, and neurological emergencies. Defibrillators, bronchodilators, epinephrine, and glucose didn't necessarily eliminate the need for hospitalization, but often stabilized patients to the point where hospitals could focus on chronic conditions underlying acute presentations.

The 70s were an important decision point for EMS: Were ambulances still primarily transport vehicles, or should they be enhanced to offer care equivalent, in many cases, to what patients would receive in ERs? It's pretty obvious we chose the latter. To what end?

There's a ton of research questioning the value of prehospital advanced life support, and just as much showing the importance of basic life support applied skillfully and promptly. What if medicine is so complex that no amount of upgrading EMS curricula will produce outcomes more favorable than prompt transport of patients to hospitals, accompanied by citizen caregivers with much less training than today's paramedics? Perhaps volunteering isn't an impediment to paid personnel, but rather the best fit for EMS.

There's a growing sentiment that volunteers are harder to find because they have less discretionary time than 20 or 30 years ago. The theory is that prospective volunteers are working more to pay for necessities.

I don't agree. It's not necessities we're working longer hours for; it's grown-up toys. We seek bigger houses, fancier cars, and more expensive vacations than our parents because we feel we deserve those things. I'm not sure when or why that sense of entitlement became prevalent, but I think it's hampering volunteering.

Another obstacle to recruitment is the burgeoning EMS curriculum at every level from EMT to paramedic. It's a dissatisfier for citizens chasing the American Dream to spend hundreds of hours on coursework.

So how do we attract post-baby-boomers to community service? Can EMS compete with consumerism? I don't have all the answers, but a first step would be to reduce the scope of EMS. The 800-hour curriculum I suggested in last month's column would help transition from today's paramedics-as-physician-extenders to "super EMTs"— more technicians than practitioners. Depending on results, we might want to cut those hours even further and empower volunteers not only with recognition and a sense of belonging, but also with less competition from, and comparison to, paid providers.

I know how crazy this all sounds. I made my living in EMS for a long time. I've known many colleagues who've helped lots of patients. I just don't see healthcare of the future embracing prehospital paraprofessionals who neither have nor desire the education of physician assistants or nurse practitioners.

Maybe it's time we moved in the opposite direction and sought semi-skilled volunteers to accompany and occasionally treat patients, but mostly to monitor them until appropriately trained professionals take over.

THE GODFATHER'S RULES FOR EMS

2015

Anyone know what day December 25th is, besides Christmas? This year it's the 25th anniversary of the release of *The Godfather Part III*, the third installment of a Hollywood epic so compelling, so majestic, so *fantastico*, the saga requires Roman numerals instead of ordinary digits for its chapters. Only a *pezzonovante* would call it *The Godfather* Part 3.

Given the early-'70s release of the first two parts and the body counts in each, the *Godfather* franchise may be partly responsible for the development of EMS in this country, and probably in Italy, too. I think I even remember an episode of *Emergency!* when Roy had to remind Johnny, "We don't discuss business at the dinner table." You have to admit, Johnny could be a little *pazzo* sometimes.

Most men I know like *The Godfather*, while most women I know like other things. I love *The Godfather*. Parts I and II are my favorite movies of all time—not that I have anything against Part III . . . well, except maybe the way Sofia Coppola, the Godfather's daughter in the movie and the director's daughter in real life, tries to keep up with actors who actually have some training. Hey, if my name were Mike Mantooth, I probably wouldn't have had to follow the same protocols as the rest of you.

Tom Hanks called *The Godfather* "the sum of all wisdom" and "the answer to any question" in his 1998 film *You've Got Mail*. I agree and propose we pay our respect to *The Godfather* by listing the ways that movie's timeless dialogue applies to everyday EMS. First, though, we need to define two common *Godfather* terms within the context of patient care:

Family: Your industry, your agency, your partner; basically, anything you care about except your real family.

Business: Stuff that happens on the ambulance and stays on the ambulance.

Here we go:

"Leave the gun, take the cannolis." If you're into metaphors, that line is quite brilliant. It reminds us to prioritize—or maybe just to eat more cannolis.

"Make him an offer he can't refuse." This is all about compromise. Say you have a patient complaining about the hospital you're heading to. Ask him if he wants to go somewhere else—a landfill.

"Command me in all things." One way to get in good with the new medical director.

"Never tell anyone outside the family what you're thinking." Very sound advice whenever circumstances force you to consider extreme, quasi-therapeutic procedures even surgeons can't do.

"Someday, and that day might never come, I will call upon you to do a service for me." Usually whispered to a student by a practical-exam preceptor who has the power to short-circuit a career quicker than you can say, "I meant to take universal precautions."

"I didn't know until this day it was Barzini all along." Just pretend *Barzini* is Italian for *pneumonia*.

"I'm a businessman; blood is a big expense." This is wrong; blood is actually a profit center. Everyone in EMS knows that. The character who said this, Bruno Tattaglia, wasn't as smart as he thought he was, and probably wouldn't have passed his hemorrhage-control station.

"Don't ask me about my business." Often said dismissively by medics to friends or spouses. Or to plaintiffs' attorneys.

"I want you to use all your powers and all your skills..." " . . . to get me out of that bloodborne pathogens class."

"Today I settled all the family business." Either your boss finally paid the past-due rent on that fire trap he calls headquarters, or you and your partner now work for a nationwide ambulette service.

"Go to the mattresses." Get some rest between calls.

"This is the business we've chosen." What you and your coworkers keep reminding each other when it hurts to lift anything heavier than your arms.

"You broke my heart." The last thing your patient thinks as you realize her saline flush was actually a dopamine flush.

"My final offer is this: Nothing." How to negotiate with volunteers.

"It's your favorite song, Michael . . . Where are you going?" A misunderstanding I have with my family whenever they gather 'round the 8-track tape player to sing "Muskrat Love."

Merry Christmas and pass the cannolis.

THE SAFETY DANCE

2017

We can dance if we want to, we've got all your life and mine
As long as we abuse it, never gonna lose it
Everything'll work out right

—Men Without Hats, 1982

*T*he scene is safe.
How often have I said that? Never on the job, but dozens of times during practical testing, when announcing scene safety is about as meaningful as declaring world peace.

Having been both the giver and taker of EMS credentialing exams for many years, I think scripted responses like "the scene is safe" are near-worthless substitutes for nuanced actions that can't be evaluated via rote vocalization. It's like saying "the heart is fine" and bypassing EKG interpretation. What bothers me most about parroting "the scene is safe," though, isn't the dumbing-down of scene size-ups during certification; it's that these exams reinforce naïveté about safety. The scene is never safe—not to the extent skill sheets imply.

Practicing scene safety takes much more than a mantra. It begins by evaluating the characteristics of the scene. Beyond obvious risks, like gaping holes in the ground or weapons pointed at you, there are subtle signs of un-safety not easily taught in a classroom—the posture of bystanders, for example, or their tone.

Next, there's a go/no-go decision based on that evaluation. Everything, including survival of patients, is supposed to be secondary to the welfare of responders. That logic can break down, though, when caution is overwhelmed by smoke billowing from a bedroom window or bodies writhing near an unseen source of methyl ethyl death.

Stop right there: How do we even begin to address the hard choices of rescue when almost every practical test scenario begins with a contrived conclusion that the scene is safe? Substituting that perfunctory disclaimer for risk management drills misleads caregivers and trivializes the chances they take every shift.

I'm not sure whether the intent is to avoid discouraging candidates who have little risk tolerance, or to reinforce our industry's macho, only-hurts-when-I-laugh culture. Probably some of both. I do think we have to find the sweet spot between acknowledging threats and becoming overwhelmed by them.

Start in almost any ambulance, where you'll hear job-related hazards minimized or even mocked by overconfident providers, whose delusions of invincibility obscure the inherent danger of prehospital environments. That's silly, but so is the belief that prophylactic procedures and protective equipment nearly eliminate risk. We shouldn't suggest, especially to our less-experienced people, that doorway surveys, sharps containers, gloves, goggles, radios, self-defense classes, ballistic vests, or chemical restraints reduce the perils of street medicine to levels of conventional jobs—the kind where you work in a climate-controlled building with offices, running water, and colleagues who are too polite to punch you.

This might be a good time to add that not all risks in EMS are physical. Some are mental, as in not necessarily leaving the field with as much faith in humans as when you entered. That doesn't mean you're a basket case when you get out; just that there are psychological issues some of us deal with after spending years serving a customer base that is simultaneously needy and unpredictable. It's okay to buy into that without ever becoming dysfunctional.

What we need is more dialogue about risk tolerance. The headline for EMS wannabes and novices should be there's no shame in deciding this field isn't for them. What isn't acceptable is trying to avoid risk altogether by shortcutting patient care—leaving the drugs and monitor on the truck at a cardiac scene to reduce back strain, for example. Joining EMS might not make you more willing to help people than the average citizen, but it shouldn't make you *less* willing, either.

We also need to stop this safety dance we do during exams. Abolish *The scene is safe* and either broaden test scenarios to include more meaningful assessments of safety or eliminate the pretense of teaching risk management. Why evaluate students on skills we're not even covering?

If I could insert a caveat into chapter one of every primary EMS textbook, it would be this: Prehospital care is physically and mentally demanding. Simply coming to work every day won't make you strong. Work out, get enough sleep, wash your hands, get your shots, find a happy place away from the job, but understand you'll still face more of a challenge to stay healthy than desk-bound workers. Meanwhile, call EMS what it is: an unsafe occupation that's not for everyone.

Author's Note

Risks to EMTs and paramedics have become even greater due to threats of violence against members of uniformed services. Self-defense classes and ballistic vests aren't substitutes for situational awareness—something I wouldn't know how to teach.

I GET YOU, BABE

2014

This column should be appearing one day after my second wedding anniversary—that's right, the anniversary of my second wedding. I think I'm finally getting the hang of it, but it might never have happened if The Lovely Helen hadn't been so assertive. I'm one of those lucky guys who actually got proposed to instead of the other way around.

I still remember that September morning in 2004 when Helen told me she had something important to discuss and said it would go better if I put down my newspaper. Then she asked, in fluent Flatbush, "You wanna get married or what?"

Unambiguous and direct—just like in the field, when she'd remind me we'd get to the hospital sooner if we actually moved patients to ambulances.

Helen was my EMS partner for eight years—a prenuptial trial I believe was no less predictive of our marriage's staying power than living together. Like marriage, EMS promotes either teamwork or conflict, depending on participants' willingness to subordinate personal wants to mutual interests. If you think that's a no-brainer, start with a simple workday test of compatibility: agreeing when and where to break for meals. If I tried to count the times my partners' cravings conflicted with my own, I'd need more fingers and toes than my species is entitled to.

Synergy in the field—shared values, common experiences, and trust—can be the basis for a relationship, but I think the odds of bonding improve when partners click on some level other than EMS. For my wife and me it was a Brooklyn connection and other generation-specific childhood memories. Also movies and music. On the way back from calls, I'd quiz Helen on famous movie lines until she'd tell me to stop doing that and play some music.

A common aspect of all my successful partnerships is that we "got" each other. I suppose that means different things to different people, but for Helen and me, it's about understanding and embracing the particulars of each personality.

Helen knows I'll probably complain about minor customer service snafus as vigorously as if our hospital gave us the wrong child; and I'm not surprised when Helen insists on doing something just because someone told her she can't. If we suddenly stopped behaving in those ways, one of us would send the other for a neurological consult.

Getting each other has practical applications in the field, like when danger is imminent. I tend to be skeptical whenever someone tells me to be careful, possibly because I never did fulfill my parents' you'll-put-out-your-eye prophecy. However, when Helen is the one doing the warning, I pay attention . . . well, usually. I trust her threat assessments because I know she and I have similar risk tolerances. I also don't want to endure second-guessing that begins with the question, "Are you mental?"

During challenging prehospital scenarios, it helps to have a partner who shares a nonverbal dialect of facial expressions and gestures. Intuitive communication saves steps and, occasionally, embarrassment. For example, there are right ways to express concern about unstable patients. None of them begin with the word *Holy*.

Even couples who get each other have issues—like the time I told Helen I'd take her out to dinner, then agreed to do one more shift; or the old girlfriend who wanted to meet me for lunch while Helen was working. Fluctuating priorities tested our relationship's staying power early on and might have prompted Helen's cautionary remark, "I don't know what I'd do without you . . . at times." But getting each other makes it easier to work through the posture-debate-consider-concede protocol during disagreements. Parties just have to guard against use of secret knowledge to intensify, rather than curtail, that process.

One sign of a successful union is asking each other, "What do you think?" and really meaning it, like when I told Helen I was writing this column and wondered how she'd characterize our 18 years as friends, partners, and spouses. In no more time than it would have taken her to check a pulse, she said, "Tell them you're a good medic, a good worker, a good father, and a halfway-decent husband."

Did I mention the importance of humor?

Author's Note

Helen and I just celebrated our 25th year of togetherness, although "celebrated" may be too kinetic a term at our ages. We had dinner and stayed up past nine.

GOOD MANNERS, BAD OUTCOME

2017

At Opryland, I worked with a paramedic we'll call Max. It took me a while to feel at ease around him, but once we got past the requisite small talk and started relating to each other, I began to think of him as a decent, conscientious guy with an OCD streak like mine. Hey, checking angiocath expiration dates together still counts as bonding.

About four years ago, Max worked an evening shift on our showboat, The General Jackson, and was scheduled to return in the morning for the day cruise. He never made it. Sometime between midnight and 10:00 AM, Max killed himself. None of us who'd served with him saw it coming. He left no note. He'd been dealing with a family issue, but appeared neither erratic nor despondent. The 38-year-old father of two was quietly confident in his abilities and evidently comfortable as part of our EMS team.

I wasn't as close to him as some of our staff were; still, I wondered what distress signals from Max I may have missed. To me, he seemed okay—more of an introvert than an extrovert and maybe even a bit shy, but those of us without the chatty gene aren't any less happy than the rest of you. Just don't leave us alone at cocktail parties.

Not everyone goes public with their darkest thoughts, despite the emergence of digital media as self-satisfying extensions of familiarity to several million significant others. For example, many in my generation—those who were raised in the 50s on a diet of do it yourself—are reluctant to let anyone know what we're feeling. It's not that we don't trust people; we just don't think you'd be terribly interested—nor should you be—in whatever is making today seem worse than yesterday in our own, tiny biospheres.

Max was born long after *strong* and *silent* were role-model criteria. What if reticence wasn't natural for him? What if it was a hint Max was pretty far from okay?

It's hard for me to imagine Max's desperation. I don't know what I'd do if I ever felt that way. My wonderful wife would want me to talk about it. Would I confess such vulnerability to her? I'd probably just keep looking for a solution on my own, but who knows? Hopelessness is so much easier to deal with when it's hypothetical.

Does the decision to end one's life bring relief? If so, is it possible to postpone the act indefinitely; to take comfort in knowing you're ready to do it without rushing into it? I'm asking because there might have been a better outcome for Max if any of us who worked with him had been less concerned about minding our manners and more inquisitive about his life away from EMS. I don't see myself being bold enough to meddle, unless . . . What if I were as pushy with Max as I am with patients? Being nosey is practically a prerequisite for paramedics. How often have I asked strangers whom I've known for 30 seconds if they're doing drugs? That certainly qualifies as getting personal.

Max needed someone to do that—to pry and not give up easily. But among 11 of us working with Max at Opryland, not one was that tenacious. What happened to our collective index of suspicion? I mean, when we ask a liquor-soiled victim of a fall if he's had anything to drink and he says no, we don't assume he was pushed.

We should have paid more attention to Max. We should have asked for more details about his home life. We weren't indifferent; we were just too polite.

Max is long past being helped, but I'd like to think I've learned a couple of lessons from that tragedy: I shouldn't assume members of generations after mine have McCarthy-era coping skills, no matter how self-sufficient they seem. And when a colleague casually mentions a potentially life-altering dilemma, I shouldn't merely echo his apparent nonchalance, but instead borrow some of the same mental-wellness assessment skills I reserve for patients. All I'd be risking is intrusiveness—not the biggest sin.

Meanwhile, in the U.S. alone there are three or four Maxes who won't show up for work tomorrow.

Reference

LiKamWa, Wendy, Erica Spies, Deborah M. Stone, Colby N. Lokey, Aimée-Rika T. Trudeau, and Brad Bartholow. "Suicide Rates by Occupational Group—17 States, 2012." *Morbidity and Mortality Weekly Report,* 65 (2016): 641–645.

HAPPY PONGAL!

January 14th is Thanksgiving in southern India—well, sort of. It's more of an agricultural festival known as Pongal. Instead of turkey, a traditional rice dish is served to celebrate a successful harvest. I mention this only because I missed an ideal opportunity in November to thank members of EMS and other essential services for helping to keep me and my patients safe for another year. So, in honor of Pongal:

To Dispatchers

I like dispatchers so much, I married one. Helen is absolutely committed to the safety of the police, fire, and EMS personnel she directs. She won't even speak to me if she has anyone on the road.

Most dispatchers I know take pride in matching resources to emergent needs. They work in dynamic, unforgiving environments where a missed transmission or wrong address can jeopardize lives. Dispatchers have been my lifeline whenever my reach has exceeded my grasp.

To Medical Control

As a new medic, I viewed medical control as just another regulatory agency that existed to micro-manage policy. I overlooked the resources they offered . . . until the first time I needed help with an ambiguous presenting problem. What a relief to discover there were no black marks appended to my name just for seeking a second opinion. Years later, when I was invited to supervise medical control for a large suburban EMS system, I vowed to offer that same level of service to new providers.

Like dispatchers, medical control personnel are constrained by not being on scene. They need superior communication skills and the talent to visualize evolving scenarios. I know I haven't always delivered the sort of presentations that make their jobs easier, but I'm grateful for their ability to bridge the gap between MDs and EMT-Ps.

To Police Officers

The thing I appreciate most about the police is that almost every time I've needed them, they've known that before I did.

Sometimes I forget I'm not a big person, and the only weapon I carry is a radio that keeps getting smaller. I could tell you stories about highly effective tactics used by men in blue to subdue scary people who wanted to make me a patient. Instead, let me just marvel at what their training and courage can accomplish in difficult situations.

Of course, police officers aren't just about protection. Some of the best first responders I've worked with have been cops. Answering "aided" calls is a natural extension of services they provide. They frequently arrive first, they're experts at scene size-up, they can enforce some degree of order amidst chaos, and they're extra hands for managing patient care and equipment. I've often thought a police officer with a paramedic card is an ideal combination of skills for the streets.

To Firefighters

The rivalry between fire and EMS is understandable, given our comparable missions, job stresses, and budget constraints. The debate about whether to combine those services will linger long after I retire. I'd rather focus on how much help I've gotten from firefighters at medical scenes.

I can't remember a firefighter ever telling me something couldn't be done. During my most challenging MCIs, whenever I've asked fire for assistance, manpower and equipment have materialized almost instantaneously. I also remember being spared indignity, and perhaps even disability, by thoughtful firefighters who loaned me protective gear when vehicle windows and posts were disintegrating around me and my patients.

I've spent only one of my 17 years in EMS working for a fire department. What impressed me about that organization was respect for the chain of command, conscientiousness about training, regard for tradition, and recognition that family and friendship are essential ingredients in any stressful occupation. Those of us in EMS-only agencies might take a lesson or two from those traits.

To EMS Management

We haven't always agreed on priorities, but to paraphrase author William Safire, "Collective opinion, when crystallized, can make history."

I've appreciated the opportunity to hear and be heard, to disagree in an atmosphere of mutual respect, and to debate without allowing egos to trump issues. Thanks to you, I'm a better medic and a better manager. I won't stop trying to give you a return on your investment in me.

To My Fellow Paramedics and EMTs

I can't imagine not being part of EMS. Sure, I gripe sometimes about long hours and low pay, and dislike the daily lumbar limbering that allows me to remain vertical, but I've had one heck of a good time. As I finish each shift and ponder the latest round of risk-taking, I'm grateful to colleagues who caught my mistakes, solved critical problems, and were partners in patient care.

Author's Note

This was the first column I ever wrote for EMS World, but it sounds more like a goodbye from me. All those thank yous still apply.

MEDICS WITH GUNS

2016

Last year I was ready to write about whether paramedics should be armed. Here's what I was going to say:

> I realize reports of violence against members of our profession seem to be escalating, but equipping public servants with enough firepower to kill patients, partners, bystanders, and themselves hardly seems like a solution. I can't imagine any realistic amount of verbal instruction or scenario-based practice being sufficient to teach medics with zero law-enforcement and military experience how to perform invasive procedures with a Glock.

Then I bought a Glock.

The world seems different to me now than it did six months ago, maybe because there were over 300 shootings involving four or more victims in the U.S. during 2015. So I decided to arm myself and up the ante for anyone who might see me as prey. I'm pretty sure that's what I am to your average maniac: prey. I say that because I'm 63 and not as spry as I used to be—not that spryness or youth are much consolation in this era of random violence.

Consider the mindset of two-legged predators: Unlike the four-legged variety, they hunt to terrorize and kill, not to eat. Unless you're in the business of profiling sociopaths, though, there's no use trying to understand them—at least not with the kind of logic favored by civilized people. How these deranged creatures got that way doesn't matter when they're hunting you. Once you become a target, the consensus from the FBI and the Department of Homeland Security is to suspend disbelief, then run, hide, and fight.

How helpful is that advice for EMS providers? Not very, if you and a predator masquerading as a patient are sharing an ambulance. As noted terrorism experts Martha and the Vandellas observed, there's "nowhere to run, nowhere to hide."

That leaves fighting. There would be no choice, I suppose, but fighting with customers is a concept I still struggle with. Something about first doing no harm made me reluctant to hit back the two times patients attacked me. I was lucky, though—a lot luckier than some of the 1,210 EMS workers out of 1,780 surveyed in 2014 who were attacked in the field.

What that survey couldn't show is how many victims of workplace violence might have been better off armed. I think that would have depended on their defensive skills and mindset—ideally, a willingness to use deadly force while understanding when not to. You're not going to learn that in a four-hour class like the one I had to pass to earn a carry permit. Unless you're in law enforcement or the military, it's pretty hard to get the kind of tactical training that sticks with you. It's sort of like working or volunteering in a low-volume, low-acuity EMS system, then one day having to sort out an MCI with multiple critical patients for the first time.

Can carrying handguns be good gambles for prehospital personnel? Perhaps, but not without serious soul searching. Consider what might happen:

- You could shoot someone who would have needed much less persuading to behave.
- You could fire at a threat and hit a bystander.
- Someone could grab your weapon within the cramped confines of an ambulance and shoot you.

I could go on, but you get the idea: Lots can go wrong. On the other hand, if you carry that sidearm off duty as well, you may have an opportunity to save more lives in places like Aurora, Colorado or Bridgewater Plaza, Virginia than in your entire EMS career.

I'd feel safer on an ambulance these days than at a shopping mall or a movie theater, and I say that after two on-duty wrecks. My wife agrees. She no longer patronizes target-rich retail environments unless I'm with her, playing bodyguard. It's a bizarre, frustrating development in our otherwise conventional lives, but all we can do is adapt to a world that's very different from the one we grew up in. Part of adapting, I believe, is taking more responsibility for our own safety and perhaps even the safety of others.

Drawing a deadly weapon around lots of innocent people is different than defending yourself one-on-one against a combative patient; however, you might be the only one at a public place with a chance to prevent carnage. If you can embrace an armed-and-vigilant off-duty role backed by whatever training you can get, accompanied by a conviction to be the most tolerant, reasonable person in any group of two or more, then maybe a sidearm makes you a little more valuable to society than just a medic card does.

At least that's what I keep telling myself.

Reference

Crowe, Remle P., Jennifer J. Eggerichs, et al. "A Description of Violence towards Emergency Medical Services Professionals." Poster presentation at the annual meeting of the National Association of Emergency Medical Services Physicians, 2014.

Author's Note

Carrying a weapon on duty has become an option in some EMS systems. I'm still not sure that's a wise choice, but I understand the concern for personal safety.

CANDLE POWER

2010

My first boss south of the Mason-Dixon Line was a paramedic named Debbie. On a July morning in 2007, I discovered what a gifted caregiver she is.

We were less than an hour into an orientation spin around my new employer's entertainment complex. It was the kind of clear, dry Tennessee dawn that makes a recovering New Yorker realize he's not getting his minimum daily requirement of hydrocarbons. I was driving the Trailblazer, trying not to miss any turns while gawking at horses recycling the local greenery. After 54 years of asphalt, I was ready for this.

Our leisurely patrol of the perimeter was interrupted by a call for a male, unknown, on a turnpike bordering our property. Less than a minute later, we found our 50-ish patient sitting on a sidewalk bench. He was wearing soiled, casual clothes and carried only a trench coat—an odd accessory on this warm, sunny day. Debbie, who beat me to the patient's side, learned that "John" had walked away from a downtown halfway house with all his possessions the night before. He was tired, hungry, and having second thoughts about seeking sympathy in the suburbs.

I was certain I knew what would happen next because I'd seen it many times: eviction of the needy from one block to another. Those cases, usually accompanied by *No patient found* dispositions, should have been coded *No compassion found*. Debbie didn't settle for that. Not only did she arrange transportation for John back to his room, she bought him breakfast while waiting for the taxi. There were no protocols to cover any of this. It was as good an example as I've ever seen of service shining through the haze of policy.

It isn't always possible for us to be so charitable with time (and in Debbie's case, money). The realities of emergent care and short transports often block our efforts to do more listening and less auscultating.

Even if we extend ourselves beyond personal preferences and pedantic protocols, our patients' prognoses don't necessarily change. John, for example, was going to be just as dependent on municipal healthcare after his cab ride as before. Are we compromising productivity by allocating time and technicians to social services? What about all the other Johns out there? How would we fit their needs into a typical workday?

Perhaps I'm overthinking this. From the time we encountered John until we waved good-bye to him, there were no other alarms. If instead of offering him assistance, Debbie had simply instructed John to move along, I suppose we would have continued my tour of the grounds—not exactly a mission-critical assignment—and forfeited our chance to improve the quality of one life for one day.

Being opportunistic about helping others, despite our dissatisfaction with the status quo, must be what Confucius had in mind when he said, "It is better to light one candle than to curse the darkness." Consider how that philosophy might lead to small but worthwhile adjuncts to prehospital care:

En-route conversations with passengers instead of with partners. Patients and their families can't help but feel unwelcome during lengthy cabin-to-cab accounts of yesterday's cool calls.

More aggressive pain management, even if it helps only for a little while. I understand the concern about administering potentially dangerous meds, but can we stop the excuses about enabling drug seekers and creating paperwork?

Extra blankets and pillows to truly achieve the oft-quoted "position of comfort." At shift change, I've often inherited ambulances without a single pillow or blanket. By operating that way, we compromise patients' comfort and lose a couple of pretty good tools for splinting extremities.

Selection of "in-flight" entertainment delegated by drivers to patients. A choice of music is one way to return a little control to customers during transport.

Shared destination decisions when logistics permit.
Passengers' preferences don't necessarily compromise protocols
or policy.

Hands held—not just palpated or cannulated. A little
empathy probably helps stable patients more than that third set
of vitals.

Such courtesies often compete not with life-saving resources, but
with apathy and inconvenience. Patients like John present fresh opportunities to make tiny improvements in the human condition. If I
put aside my clipboard and concentrate on little things that matter, I
might just find a few less emergent but much appreciated services to
offer my patients.

The holidays are near. What better time to light a candle?

SHARING THE BURDEN

2010

The first thing a visitor notices outside the Shanksville, Pennsylvania Volunteer Fire Department is the 12-foot-high steel cross adorning the front lawn. How odd that a religious icon would decorate a municipal agency in this age of acute political correctness.

The giant cross is a gift from New York City's Fire Family Transport Foundation. The vertical and horizontal beams are worn and warped, just as they were when they were pulled from a five-story, 16-acre pile that had been the World Trade Center. Delivered by that city's fire department (FDNY) in 2008, then mounted on a pentangular base, the structure is a reminder that there were not one, nor two, but three grounds zero on 9/11. Shanksville Chief Terry Shaffer inherited the third.

Shaffer was one of millions of Americans that morning watching miscreants use commandeered jetliners to slaughter thousands in massive structures thought to be impregnable. Like most of us, Terry's reaction was buffered by distance and disbelief.

"Are you aware of what's going on?" his wife called him at work to ask. Shaffer assumed she meant the carnage in New York and Washington and assured her he was following the news.

"Well, you have a plane down in your district and you need to come home right now."

Terry thought she was joking or he'd misunderstood her, because there were no other conceivable scenarios. He called a dispatcher for confirmation, then raced from Johnstown to the crash site, 80 miles southeast of Pittsburgh. Forty minutes after United Airlines Flight 93, inverted and ballistic, struck an abandoned strip mine two miles from the Shanksville-Stonycreek School, Chief Shaffer stood at a 50-foot crater made by the fuel-laden Boeing 757 traveling at Mach .74.

"There was debris everywhere," Shaffer recalls. "Lots of wiring and thousands of pieces no bigger than my fist. The only things that looked like airplane parts were a turbine and some tires. You could smell jet fuel and burnt flesh."

It was evident to all who responded—fire, EMS, police—that their mission would be recovery, not rescue. Somerset County Coroner Wally Miller spotted just one body part—a length of spine with five vertebrae—during his initial walk-through. Miller subsequently identified all 37 passengers, including four hijackers, and seven crewmembers from 1,500 discrete human remains weighing approximately 600 pounds—only 8% of the theoretical total. The rest had likely vaporized on impact.

Shanksville's firefighters, ten of whom are EMTs, extinguished brush fires and helped the state police clear bystanders from what would be Pennsylvania's longest active crime scene, then spent three weeks with FEMA and the FBI salvaging fragments of the plane and its passengers. Terry had concerns about the emotional toll on his people. "I tried to restrict access to those who had been on-site since the beginning," he says, "but that was pretty naïve on my part." (Counseling, offered early and often, has helped Shanksville retain 75% of its members from nine years ago.)

The most prominent reminder of the disaster in this tiny borough of 245 residents is the Flight 93 National Memorial adjacent to the field where the airliner disintegrated. An unobstructed view from the gallery reveals no evidence of the catastrophe—no scorched earth, no severed trees, no scattered debris. The only landmark, barely visible hundreds of yards away, is an American flag draped over a fence post. That is where all but the most forward segments of the 155-foot-long jet burrowed into the ground. That is also where 40 passengers and crewmembers, responding to the ultimate airborne emergency, suffered the consequences of their selflessness.

It's as hard to imagine wreckage smoldering in the pristine pastures of Shanksville as in the urban fortresses of New York City and Washington, DC. Processing the horrific, even when buttressed by bravado, is universally traumatic. There's only one level of unimaginable.

"I don't think anyone could train for an event of this magnitude," Shaffer says, "but I think we stepped up to the plate, had help from lots of other departments, and displayed the kind of professionalism you'd want from both paid and volunteer services."

Shaffer credits his ongoing relationships with New York and DC rescuers for a healthy post-9/11 perspective. "I feel really close to those people. It may be a cliché, but we're all brothers."

The Shanksville cross symbolizes that fellowship. It reminds us disaster is an uncompromising equalizer. When mortals and metal fall from the sky, distinctions between fire and EMS, big and small, urban and rural, BLS and ALS, paid and volunteer, matter little. Those who respond and survive are tormented by what they tried to do, had to do, couldn't do. We share their burden as brethren.

Author's Note

A permanent memorial to the passengers and crew of United Flight 93 was dedicated in Shanksville a year after I wrote this column.

THE EMS BOOK CLUB

2010

My daughter, Becky, has been fascinated by all things medical since she watched her father's tentative steps toward an EMS career 18 years ago. For her birthday last month, I wanted to buy her a book about prehospital care that's informative, well-written, up-to-date, irreverent, entertaining, and not too technical—the EMS equivalent of, say, *Kitchen Confidential* by Anthony Bourdain, without the references to edible body parts.

I couldn't find any non-fiction that met my criteria, not that there's anything wrong with the authors out there. I just think we need a source specializing in off-beat EMS literature—books that expose the underbelly of our profession while reminding us it's okay to laugh at things like projectile vomiting, particularly when the recipient is wearing a suit during a ride-along.

Relax, I've got it covered. Here are six cutting-edge publications I've chosen for my very own, soon-to-be-financed-by-reverse-mortgages EMS book club. Let me know if any of these interest you. Operators are standing by, somewhere.

I'm a Real Medic and You're Not

Forget all those life-in-the-streets tearjerkers—the ones written by "bleeding hearts" about bleeding hearts. *I'm a Real Medic and You're Not* targets EMS wannabes who prefer insults to insight. The author, a practicing microcephalic, warns that anyone willing to buy his book is, by definition, incapable of understanding the subtleties of it. Only those licensed before the Boer War are senior enough to fit the author's criteria for real medics.

The One-Minute Checkout

Tired of checklists? Want more time to sit around and complain about low pay, frequent flyers, unsympathetic spouses, psychotic partners, and pets that eat furniture? If so, *The One-Minute Checkout* is for you. Here are just a few of the labor-saving shortcuts you'll learn:

- Fine-tune your "oxygen awareness." Does that D tank *look* full? Then it probably is.
- Don't worry about checking drugs you hardly ever use. You've probably forgotten the dosages, anyway.
- Don't be too quick to fuel your rig. Gasoline is expensive.
- Cardiac monitors are a lot lighter without batteries. Just remember to carry a few old EKGs in case someone asks for one.

Pass Paramedic! And Geometry!

It is an impressive compilation of scenarios that pay homage to both Hippocrates and Euclid. According to the publisher, students who read all 18,196 square inches of this text are 3.1415926 times more likely to pass their EMT-P and GED exams. Here's a sample:

You're called to the scene of a patient struck by a rhombus. Your first action would be:

a. Control bleeding with a rectangular dressing.
b. Immobilize the patient on an elliptical backboard.
c. Open the airway by rotating the mandible 17 degrees through an arc with a four-foot radius.
d. Report "no patient found" and go have a square meal.

The answer is d because a rhombus is a two-dimensional shape that can't hurt you unless you're a cartoon character.

Schlegel's Book of Silly EKGs

In this case-oriented offering, Dr. Schlegel discusses some of the strangest electrocardiograms he's encountered and his creative approach to cardiac care. Readers are invited to anticipate Schlegel's interventions when, for example, he spots Wandering Accelerated T-waves (rapid infusion of conducting gel followed by a prayer vigil) or Left-Right Ventricular Shift (call 9-1-1, then discourage breathing).

Great War Stories of the Twentieth Century

This comprehensive, entertaining anthology is best suited for folks who attend *Third Watch* conventions or have at least one pet named Rampart. Tales of dangling and mangling are divided into chapters such as "Power Tools for Venous Access," "High-Angle Intubation," and "Treating Hypotension with Reinfused Flashback."

10,001 Practice Questions for EMT Entrance Exams

There are plenty of EMS workbooks out there, but only one devoted to that first big step: admission to an EMT course. Rather than follow the customary multiple-choice-question-and-answer approach, the editors save time and space by omitting both the multiple choices and answers. The result is a simplified study guide that will appeal primarily to existentialists. Here are a few questions:

1. *I have two pagers and you have three pagers. Which one of us has two pagers?*
2. *If Dick and Jane leave headquarters at the same time, when will they return?*
3. *When did Congress pass the Highway Safety Act of 1966?*
4. *What's your favorite bone, and why?*

Other books available:

*   *Things Doctors Order*
*   *Chest Tubes for Dummies*

- *Man Down! 'Cause We Dropped Him!*
- *The Observer's Guide to Being of No Consequence*
- *God Is My Flashlight*
- *ESM for Dyslexics*

Author's Note

I actually got two book orders from readers. Explaining the joke to them was not fun.

CRITICAL CARE

2009

Some calls stay with us longer than others. You know what I mean. My patient was a 50-ish female complaining of . . . well, she wasn't really complaining about anything. I found her contracted in bed with animated eyes and a sly smile. I learned from her daughter that mom had spina bifida and was in constant pain. She also seemed to be a little short of breath. When I announced after a brief exam that her fever and congestion could be signs of pneumonia, my patient said she would gladly tolerate any illness responsible for attracting such a handsome man to her bedroom.

I think she caught me looking around for a handsome man. She tugged at my hand to regain my attention, then told me I reminded her of her late husband, except he wasn't bald. Her mischievous expression dissolved during a coughing fit, but returned when I promised to carry her from her bed to our stretcher. As I lifted her scoliotic frame, she asked if that meant we were engaged.

I transported her a second time after her illness had progressed. We indulged in the same playful banter just days before she died. I learned of the outcome when her daughter and I nearly sideswiped each other's shopping carts in a supermarket several months later. I was surprised at how many details I remembered about her mother. It took me a while to figure out why: She was the first patient I'd connected with on more than a professional level.

I spent the first two years after medic school trying to master the science of our profession. I'm not sure I succeeded, or ever will, but I did develop a systematic approach to prehospital care that kept me out of trouble. By Year 3 I was pretty comfortable with everything we carried on our ambulances—except patients. I wasn't the most sociable medic and found small talk distracting. Senior colleagues mostly validated my perspective by encouraging me to focus on procedures, not people.

One partner who, to minimize inconvenience, had culled a personal subset of standing orders from our protocols, dismissed administration of analgesics because "we're not the ones in pain." That contributed to my view of EMS as a soulless, process-driven vocation not very different from the manufacturing sector I'd left behind.

My impish patient helped dispel that gloomy image. At first, as she disarmed me with her droll remarks, I resisted turning our dialogue into something informal. I didn't want pleasantries to get in the way of my routine. En route to the hospital, though, I discovered I enjoyed her company, and sensed her well-being had less to do with needles and drugs than with our conversation. Other than monitoring vitals and providing comfort, all I did was listen to her and sometimes respond. Care was secondary to caring—a new concept for me that seemed to work for both of us.

Do feelings interfere with performance? Many of my colleagues would respond affirmatively. The "John Wayne" culture of essential services discourages emotion. Expressions of empathy for patients are often regarded as weaknesses to be wrung out of providers during primary training. Failure to recognize a middle ground between ineffectual sentimentality and robotic behavior leads to reinforcement of the Spartan self-image some of us cultivate. We are beginning to understand, however, that stoicism is less healthy than prompt, informal discussion of acute stressors with family and friends.

None of the people I know who resigned after years of unhappiness in EMS blamed "caring too much" for their career change. Quite the opposite: Most of them complained of apathy accompanied by a sense of hopelessness. Perhaps a more robust support structure would have reassured them that they still could make a difference, one patient at a time.

It would be naïve to portray all our customers as selfless romantics who see us as their spiritual guides. Some merely want the facts—and maybe a sliver of speculation—about their medical conditions. We're not doctors, but we can offer patients abridged versions of differentials, prognoses, and treatment options. Staying current in our field to answer such technical questions is another way of caring.

Like most of you I've had bad days in EMS, but I don't think any of them were caused by paying too much attention to my patients. I do regret not caring more about some. Perhaps I didn't know how.

Sometimes it was hard to summon emotions as peers reinforced an ambivalent, just-another-job mentality. Besides, I had to get past my own protocol-driven agenda and consider whether my patient of the moment might be better served by empathy and eye contact than scripted procedures.

Two-thirds of a career later, I'm willing to admit I went to the funeral of that frail patient with the fun-loving demeanor. The memories I shared with her family didn't render me non-functional, nor did they make me contemplate an alternative career path. Instead, I felt empowered by my acceptance of compassion as beneficial, rather than detrimental, to prehospital practice. I like myself better this way.

Sometimes we just need to find reasons to care.

COACH CLASS

2012

A few months ago, I swapped emails with Paul, a close friend and ex-partner from New York. Paul and I are in the autumns of our EMS careers—early December, I'd say. We were discussing how hard it will be to leave. Is it possible, we wondered, to find another activity as stimulating as prehospital care, but without the physical challenges made even more formidable by age?

After reading "Personal Best," Atul Gawande's compelling piece about coaching in the Oct. 3, 2011 issue of *The New Yorker*, I think I might have an answer. Gawande, a surgeon, discussed the benefits of inviting a respected retired instructor to monitor his cases. Gawande claims that process—live observation of technique followed by debriefing, critique, and forward-looking strategy sessions—lowered his complications rate and reinvigorated his practice.

Is there a need for coaching in EMS beyond certification-driven objectives? I think so. I know I would have been sharper with periodic, practical tune-ups that went beyond review of the same skill sheets I'd mastered two or three years before. Even today, after almost 20 years in this industry, I'm sure there are aspects of my performance that could be improved through impartial observation by an experienced associate, followed by customized feedback.

Some would say EMS already provides coaches. They're called preceptors or field training officers (FTOs). I disagree. Those titles imply senior-junior or teacher-student hierarchies. Newbies rarely get to pick their FTOs, nor do they have a say in the goals or the scope of that interaction. Coaching veteran providers requires a different skill set than guiding novices through their earliest field interventions. For example, a good coach might lack limitless patience for rookie mistakes, while a good preceptor might find it hard to offer advice constructively and diplomatically to a coworker with as much or more experience.

Consider those who carry the title *coach* in sports; they haven't necessarily performed as long or as well as their charges. With so many media outlets competing for the attention of the coachable, I think modern coaches need exceptional communication skills more than been-there-done-that pedigrees. That's fortunate for me, because I've never done a cric with a car key or started a central line in an elevator shaft.

Is coaching equivalent to mentoring? Similar, perhaps, but not the same. Coaching involves direct, ongoing oversight with real-time guidance. Mentoring is more of a passive activity without mandate or even mention. I can imagine asking a trusted colleague to be my coach, but not my mentor. I doubt any of the mentors I've had in journalism, sports, engineering, or EMS knew they were playing that role.

A prerequisite to coaching is someone who wants to be coached. That might be trickier than it sounds. To those of you with more than a few years in this field, how willing are you to endure scrutiny and criticism of your work habits? Could you consider suggestions impersonally in the spirit of well-intended quality improvement? Sometimes that's hard for me, even when I know my patients or readers or clients would be the beneficiaries. My first reaction to recommendations is often "Yes, but . . ." If I were coaching me, I'd put a stop to that.

Here's what I'd want from a coach:

Distinguish style from substance. Doing things my way isn't necessarily wrong; however, I'm willing to try almost anything to improve my performance that doesn't lead to a court appearance or a viral YouTube video.

Don't limit feedback to what you think I want to hear. I already know enough people who do that. I'm not saying I don't like it sometimes; I just think positive reinforcement means a lot more when it's balanced by constructive negatives.

Be of service. Your job is to help me. If you're good at that, you'll meet your needs by sincerely addressing mine.

I wouldn't be surprised if many retired EMTs and medics met those criteria. They're occupational skills. We don't forget how to do those things just because we're on the sidelines. I hope I can leverage my share of life experience to help others in EMS long after my last paycheck.

Come see me in a few years. I'll be the one with the patch that says *Coach.*

Author's Note

This idea hasn't gained any traction. I suppose writing is a form of coaching, but it lacks the one-on-one guidance I had in mind.

CERTIFICATION EXPERIMENTATION

2015

This might be just another March for you. For me, it marks a big step in my eventual return to civilian life.

Take a look at my bio; this is the last time you'll see *NR* after my name. The National Registry requires members to be active practitioners —like with protocols and medical direction and stethoscopes. I still have my ears somewhere, but that's about it. I haven't treated a patient since 2013.

I thought maybe I could get certified as the EMS World house medic, but my editor says there's a law against her signing *MD* after her name. Yup, even in California. I told her she could always say MD stands for Master of Deadlines or Memorized Dictionary—especially in California. She said something about me having an omega-3 deficiency and invited me to do a feature on résumé-writing.

Next, I wondered if I could get an EMS job somewhere that doesn't involve bending, squatting, and lifting. A Google search came up with two possibilities: paramedic on a merry-go-round and night-shift medic at a cemetery. If the latter comes with cable and a Barcalounger, I'm interested.

The Registry says *EMT-P* is being phased out, so I'm wondering what I should call myself after March 31st. If I were still registered, it would be)*NRP*, per Registry guidelines for paramedics. Does that mean I'll be *NNRP*, as in *not* nationally registered, after 3/31?

I could accentuate the positive and call myself *state*-registered, or *SRP*, except that sounds like there should be a price after my name. What if I drop the *S* and make it *RP* for *registered paramedic*? Is *RP* any better than just plain *P*? Yeah, I know, several words starting with *P* fit me. We'll go through those some other time.

I could always settle for *Mike Rubin, paramedic.* Sounds a little pretentious, though. Even in Hollywood, where embellishment is a way of life, *Marcus Welby, Doctor* would have been a bit much.

Back to that idea about state registry: I'm still a Tennessee paramedic. I even have a license that says so. The Volunteer State has pretty much bet the ranch I won't do anything heroic and stupid to patients in the name of Davy Crockett or Alvin York. I appreciate Tennessee's loyalty and would like to acknowledge their commitment to me by substituting *TN* for *NR*, as in *TNP.* Wherever I go, whatever I do, everyone will know where my medical direction is supposed to be coming from.

Couldn't all medics who aren't nationally registered use their state abbreviations followed by *P*? Right away we'd be identifying our state, our protocols, and which side we were on in the 1860s. I bet some of those *nationally registered* medic-elitists would downgrade just so they could be like us; well, maybe not too many. Still, it would be cool to be part of a brand-new trend that doesn't involve ballistic vests.

Adding state abbreviations would create some interesting acronyms. For example, Hawaii would be a good place for medics my age to work, not only because of the climate and scenery, but because we'd all finally be *HIP.* I spent a lot of time trying to be hip in the 60s. I'm not sure I ever made it. I had the Nehru jacket, but the medallion was too heavy and expensive. When the Hollies sang "He ain't heavy," they definitely weren't talking about someone with a medallion.

Colorado would be popular with medics who got into EMS only because they failed law-enforcement physicals. There's something exhilarating about becoming a *COP* without any training. You're basically telling the world you're a freethinker—an individualist not constrained by other people's rules, except the ones recommending incarceration for police impersonators.

Do they have medics in the Virgin Islands? They must, at least for sunburns and jellyfish stings, right? Well, then we finally have a place where paramedics will get the respect we deserve. I'm talking about priority seating at the swankiest restaurants, free passes to the best shows, and courtesy detours around security checkpoints at airports, if they have any airports in the Virgin Islands. Just show your *VIP* card.

And then there's Rhode Island.

A SUBSTANCE PROBLEM

2016

How many times have you been underwhelmed by the performance of uber-hyped medical devices? I'm talking about the difference between form (the way something appears) and substance (how well it works). That gap gets real pretty fast in the field.

EMS is supposed to be all about substance. One of my preceptors told me that. Or maybe he said "substances." That's another column. Meanwhile, form influences EMS providers way more than it should. We develop preferences for brands and designs often without knowing why.

Sometimes we're imagining a solution to a problem that doesn't exist, like a "CPR seat" in the back of an ambulance I used to ride. That add-on seemed like a great idea until we realized its location made it useful only if the AHA promoted pelvic compressions.

Other times, form in one environment doesn't translate well to a different setting. Crisp, white button-down shirts with pockets, epaulets, and insignias are good examples. They look so professional on scene until the inevitable splotches of grease and blood deface them within a day of laundering. Such dressy clothes for dirty jobs belong in the era when filling-station attendants wore bow ties.

Then there's the stuff that just looks cool, like the pouches I used to wear on my belt before I realized most of what I needed on calls was between my ears. Yes, I said *pouches*, as in more than one at a time. I carried two pairs of scissors, umbilical clamps, tweezers and a bite stick in one. I'm not sure why; maybe they came as a package. The other pouch had an EMS field guide, trauma shears, hemostats and a scalpel. Doctors who hung out with me would have had everything they needed to perform a C-section on a seizing patient with ticks.

My personal-best case of form over substance in EMS was a "rolling tourniquet" I bought after going through a streak of blown IVs. The device was essentially a nine-inch-long spring wrapped in a soft, white sheath with plastic clasps at either end. The idea was to bind the tourniquet around an arm proximal to an IV site, then roll the contraption distally to milk blood into the target vein. That worked well if the limb was the right size for the tourniquet. Any skinnier and there'd be no milking; any fatter and the tourniquet would hurt more than the IV.

The vendor's solution was to offer two other sizes: large and small. Once you owned all three tourniquets, you could even combine them to accommodate almost any arm's circumference. Or you could just do the IV the way you were taught.

The substance problem isn't limited to EMS. In the '80s, I had a car that came with an inclinometer—a gauge that told me how far we were leaning left or right. Sitting on top of the dashboard, it made an otherwise-ordinary console look like a cockpit. Sweet!

The driver's manual didn't have much to say about the inclinometer—only that if the needle goes past 45 degrees, you're already tipping over. Good to know if you drive sideways along the White Cliffs of Dover.

It's easy to be seduced by form. Substance isn't as obvious, as it waits to be discovered by customers who insist on nothing less than practicality. Sometimes you have to dig through elaborate packaging to find value, because form is what gets products sold. Substance gets them used.

Here are my favorite instances of substance over form in the field:

- **Glucometers:** They absolutely changed the way we handled AMS cases in the mid-'90s.
- **Pulse oximeters:** The initial argument against them was that they weren't needed to diagnose hypoxemia, but they became standard of care and were eventually built into cardiac monitors.
- **Capnometry:** These devices took off when clunky, analog units were replaced by in-line digital readouts.
- **Smartphones:** Suddenly everything you needed to know about meds, diseases, and how to say "chest pain" in 18 Indo-European languages was accessible real-time.

If you're looking for something less mainstream, consider carrying a large paper clip that can be elongated and attached to an IV bag at one end and a curtain at the other. Or use one of those fancy hemostats I mentioned to do the same.

What's the next frontier in EMS for form over substance? Miniaturization, I hope. Think how much easier your job would be if monitors and radios were much smaller but just as functional. O_2 tanks, too; imagine "A" cylinders with "D" capacity. How about BVMs that aren't so klutzy? And smaller IV bags with desiccated saline that hydrates when squeezed. These are ideas waiting for someone smarter than me to implement.

If it's cool toys you prefer, I can make you a deal on rolling tourniquets in three handy sizes.

Author's Note

I went searching for those rolling tourniquets in the Rubin Museum of Leftover EMS Stuff. No joy, but I did find BDUs that used to fit someone much thinner.

DESK DUTY

2013

Early this year I met The Lovely Helen for dinner after my Opryland shift. I remember complaining about not having a chance to change clothes (to which Helen countered, "At least *I* look good."). I didn't realize I'd wear that uniform only once more.

My July paycheck was probably my last as an EMS provider. I decided it was time to leave Opryland after I had difficulty assuming and maintaining a crouched position while treating a patient with rapid a-fib in a cramped space. I got through the call, but I realized I could no longer do my job safely. My back was holding me back.

This isn't a sob story about disability disrupting a promising career. I'm 60. I started working when gasoline cost 30 cents a gallon. I was in grade school when Eisenhower was president. The one before Kennedy.

The baggers at my local supermarket know I'm old, not just because of the gray in my beard: This year I started getting a senior discount. I wasn't going to sign up for that privilege until I got *really* old—say, 62—but then I figured it would help me save for Depends. Funny how you never really finish buying diapers.

Although I joined the AARP 10 years ago, I'm not retiring. I plan to stay involved in EMS by writing about it and sometimes needing it. I'll be working from my desk—the one I'm standing at right now. Standing is more comfortable for me than sitting. I find I write better when I'm comfortable, which works against the whole struggling-writer-bares-his-soul syndrome. I'm hoping to avoid the equally compelling intoxicated-writer-bares-his-soul syndrome.

What I won't be doing is sitting around watching TV. There's nothing more dispiriting than daytime television. When I was a kid, midday TV meant quiz shows and soap operas. You only watched those if you were home sick. Even now, when someone mentions

Guiding Light or *As The World Turns*, I feel sick. *The Jerry Springer Show* has the same effect on me, but for different reasons.

I'm a big fan of EMS. I've felt that way since my first call two decades ago. I'm sure I've frustrated many partners who've tried to convince me our jobs suck. Sometimes they do, but I've been happier with EMS than any of the other 11 occupations I've tried. Even on bad days, I figured there was a chance things would get better on the next call. Often, they did.

I have so many good memories of being in the field, it would be hard to choose the best. All of these would make the top 10:

- I answered my first EMS call—a minor industrial accident— soon after I started volunteering in New York. I remember being encouraged by the EMT in charge to apply my first-aid training. Turns out that stuff worked on real patients. Thank you, Sally.
- A year later, I became an EMT. Although I was 40 and had been fairly successful in business, I don't think I'd ever felt as proud as I did when I got my fist card in the mail. I was ready to save the world, one chief complaint at a time. My instructor had a lot to do with that enthusiasm. Thank you, Reeve.
- My goal after graduating medic school 18 months later was to learn my trade in New York City. Good jobs were hard to find there, but one referral opened that door. It felt great to make the "majors." Thank you, Paul.
- I wore a suit to work my first day as supervisor of medical control for Suffolk County, New York, because that had been the dress code at almost all of my corporate postings. By noon I'd realized I could forget about commercial trivialities, ditch the jacket and tie, and focus on more important matters—like keeping people safe. Thank you, Eric.
- My last call came a few hours after that a-fib case I mentioned earlier. The patient had a debilitating, chronic condition we both knew was beyond treating. We sat and talked for 45 minutes. It was good for both of us. Thank you, my friend.

I'm sad I won't be making new EMS memories, but I'm thankful to have come this far without screwing up too badly. I always figured I was one big mistake away from notoriety. Perhaps that mentality helped me do better. Or maybe I was lucky. All I know is, I won't be tormented by what-ifs as I continue to write about life from a caregiver's perspective.

It was worth moving out from behind a desk for 21 years, if only to work with people like you.

Author's Note

So here I am, writing from the sidelines of EMS. It is indeed better than watching dumb TV, but I miss the kick of patient care.

DUTY TO REACT

2015

Half a century ago, 28-year-old Kitty Genovese was stalked and stabbed in New York City. I remember the case well—not because of its location or outcome, but because of a report that 38 people witnessed the crime and did nothing. Although that estimate has since been reduced to five, the Genovese murder reminds us that not getting involved can have tragic consequences.

Much more recently, an EMS forum I follow published a post from an off-duty EMT who wondered if he was right to answer a commuter-train crew's request for help with an elderly victim of a fall. The newly certified responder, who checked the passenger's pulse, took a SAMPLE history, and evaluated her according to the Cincinnati Stroke Scale, chided himself for not being able to determine the cause of her fall and questioned whether he'd helped the patient at all.

When I read his account I thought, *Good for him; here's someone new to our field who gets the part about helping others.* Then critical comments like "I probably would have just called 9-1-1" and "Don't get involved" started appearing, and I began to wonder how long it would take the ambivalence of colleagues to erode our diligent EMT's enthusiasm.

Yes, there are risks of administering care away from one's district, but I've never believed a uniform or a duty to act is the most important consideration when someone is sick or hurt. I try not to overthink the downside of good intentions; I only know I'd want others to show the same concern for members of my family in distress.

Maybe it's inconvenient and just plain bad luck to be the only one with medical training at an emergency. It's impractical and not at all fun to stop at a train wreck without gear or back-up. Discovering the freshly dead is unpleasant enough when we're on the job; dealing with the misery of serious illness or injury on a day off isn't anyone's idea of recreation.

When you're there, you're there. You can try to ignore it and keep driving while telling yourself it's someone else's territory, someone else's scene. You might even justify that attitude by reminding yourself you spent the last 24 hours answering that kind of calls, and now it's someone else's turn.

Seriously?

What if there's a delay in the 9-1-1 system? What if the responding crew lacks your training or experience? When did it become okay to bet a life with someone else's chips?

I don't think most of us entered EMS with lots of self-imposed conditions about when and how we'd engage in rescue. When I got started, I wasn't too picky about which patients I'd treat on duty or off. I was on a 24/7 safari for the elusive good call—naïve and even silly perhaps, but I wasn't about to let any opportunities to play medic pass by.

Have you ever felt that way? When did it change for you? Was it when you realized we don't make a huge difference every day—not that we don't make *any* difference, just not as much as we'd hoped? Or were you on a call so horrific, you figured the only way to survive in EMS while achieving some measure of longevity was to titrate your compassion?

I get that, but sometimes we underestimate the difference conversation, counsel, and even handholding can make to someone hurting and needy. No one had to explain that to Sophia Farrar, the only Genovese neighbor who left the safety of locked doors to offer aid. Without medical training, Farrar easily could have rationalized letting someone else be the rescuer. Instead, she focused on what she *could* do. Genovese died in her arms.

The anniversary of Kitty Genovese's murder is a sobering reminder of a population's capacity for indifference. It doesn't matter whether 38 people or five witnessed the attack; citizens who might have intervened favored refuge over rescue, convenience over care. The only contribution to society offered by most of those onlookers was clarification of the term *bystander*.

We in EMS are better than that, aren't we? When faced with distress—not even danger—don't we have a bias to intercede? We used to. *You* used to. You know who you are—the ones who set examples for me; the ones who took care of my daughter, my wife, my mother, my father. Please tell me you're still out there.

PARTNERS

2010

I'm not a big fan of prime-time EMS dramas. When they stray from "gritty realism" toward vacuous story lines favoring voodoo medicine, they make me say bad things to my TV. None of my home appliances deserve such treatment.

Shows such as *Saved* and *Third Watch* have portrayed one part of EMS pretty accurately: our mutually dependent, sometimes volatile relationships with partners. Does any aspect of our profession have a bigger impact on job satisfaction? I don't think so.

Partners can make a busy day exhilarating or a slow shift interminable. Their mere presence fosters serenity or provokes IBS. They can be conscientious, contentious, sociable, unapproachable, pragmatic, or enigmatic. The only constant about partners is that they're ours until shift change or hand-to-hand combat—whichever occurs first.

I feel fortunate to have worked beside many considerate, supportive, perceptive peers. I've also encountered a few wackos who were one psych evaluation away from the medic wing at the cracker factory. I'm thinking of the guy who barked like a schnauzer at pedestrians as we responded to alarms. Another used two hand puppets as squeaky-voiced surrogates to admonish noncompliant patients:

Left Hand: "Mike didn't take his blood pressure medicine today."

Right Hand: "Really? Why not?"

Left Hand: "Because Mike's a bad boy!"

Partnerships begin with an awkward phase that sometimes seems like weeks, but is usually just a shift or two. During that time, we're seeking compatibility and compromise. We're also figuring out the answer to a very important question: Can my partner meet my needs?

That sounds selfish, but we're just trying to find out if we can play to each other's strengths and compensate for each other's weaknesses.

I had a rocky start with IVs. After missing three during one shift as a new medic, I decided I was a threat to public safety and should limit my community service to lemonade stands. Fortunately, my next call allowed me to showcase my intubation skills while my more experienced partner started a difficult line. One successful invasive procedure boosted my confidence and encouraged me to swap roles on our next two jobs (both cardiac arrests). My partner cooperated, just as I had when he preferred to drive.

I've heard people liken partners to spouses. I disagree. EMS objectives are mostly short-term—stabilization of illness and injury en route to definitive care—rather than lifelong quests for fulfillment shared with significant others. Also, there's an element of risk in the essential services that most of us don't endure at home. Stress associated with that risk can lead to intense loyalty and an us-against-the-world mentality among partners that many couples never know.

Some EMS agencies require partners to rotate. Why interfere with partnerships that work? That's like replacing Mick Jagger with Donnie Osmond on the Stones' next tour. If there are concerns about business being compromised by personal relationships, I can only say I've witnessed more pros than cons when colleagues become close friends.

I prefer partners who bring a "we" mentality to work. Each of us is entitled to:

Vigilance. Once when I was working a code as a new medic, I grabbed Lasix instead of lidocaine. I don't know why—maybe because both start with the same letter. Perhaps I would have discovered my error before pushing the Lasix. We'll never know because my partner stopped me before I implemented a novel cardiac arrest algorithm. Division of labor during difficult calls doesn't allow us to double-check everything, but it's good to have another set of eyes. Ears, too—like when a belligerent, intoxicated patient boasts he's a mercenary and an ex-con (my benevolent intervention of the week).

Conscientiousness. Many of us supplement subsistence-level EMS wages with other income-producing activities, but we can only concentrate on one job at a time. I don't want my partner preoccupied with stock portfolios or sales calls when we should be in medic mode.

Consideration. If I'm paying the price for fusing Thai and Korean cuisine the night before, can we go easy on the jalapeños today? I promise to do the same for you. Also, music of any genre played loudly enough to induce tinnitus isn't entertaining, it's diabolical.

I think we seek different qualities in partners as we gain experience and self-sufficiency. Early in my career, I hung with the crazies because comic relief calmed my nerves. Later, as call volume became my antidote to awkwardness, I sought partners who practiced at a higher level, systematically vectoring toward working diagnoses that were almost always correct, or at least close. Even as my career winds down, I remain determined to learn from anyone who screws up less than I do.

Polished practitioners leave lasting impressions. The best partner I ever had, an EMT from the mean streets of Brooklyn, taught me EMS shouldn't be a choice between BLS and ALS, but rather a continuum of care. We worked so well together, I doubt patients suspected our levels of certification differed. Even today, that partner and I are two halves of the same whole.

Maybe that's why I married her.

Author's Note

I've made plenty of mistakes. Marrying Helen wasn't one of them.

HOW MUCH?

2014

Joey, a family member with whom I'm not on speaking terms, had a bad GI bleed a few months ago. I'm pretty sure he hates trips to the doctor as much as I do. Fortunately, Joey knows nothing about his right to consent, so I half-dragged him to the car, told him to quit complaining, tossed him in the back, and tied him to his seat. We were going to the hospital whether he liked it or not.

All you champions of the sick and helpless—chill; Joey is an eight-year-old Cavalier King Charles spaniel. He's a good dog but a bad patient, which, on a very weird level, makes us similar. Or so I've been told. More importantly, Joey is going to help me make a point about customer service.

I liked the way the veterinarian and her staff treated Joey. The receptionist asked if our dog might like a snack, then quoted a minimum charge for office visits. Next, the vet introduced herself and said she'd go over the rest of the costs after Joey's exam. That was fine with me—much better than the price gouging that sometimes follows care of two-legged patients.

That trip to the vet made me wonder why we can't do the same for *our* customers—not the part about giving them biscuits when they behave; I mean discussing pricing prehospitally. The antiquated attitude that dollars shouldn't sway treatment decisions is unrealistic in this era of sky-high deductibles. If I were a stable patient, I'd want to know about costly interventions while I still had a chance to delay or dismiss them.

I think the Affordable Care Act makes consumers more aware of healthcare costs. Suddenly, there's a marketplace where competition forces underwriters to detail prices and services. I'm not any happier with insurance premiums than I was before the ACA, but at least I know better what I'm getting for what I'm spending.

Looking at healthcare as just another service might help us understand the importance of pricing to our patients. I certainly wouldn't commit to home repairs, for example, without knowing the cost. My willingness to incur those charges would depend on the degree of damage. I wouldn't want a contractor to assume I'd pay for a new roof just because of a water stain. Even a big hole in the ceiling wouldn't change my right as a homeowner to decide what work should be done.

It's the same in EMS, where water stains could be blood and holes are, well, holes. As medical professionals, we're supposed to get informed consent from alert patients before taking action, no matter how routine or necessary treatment seems to us. The consequences to healthcare providers of making decisions without patients' involvement can be unsettling and, at worst, devastating.

I've been indirectly involved in one lengthy lawsuit alleging transport without consent. I don't know how it turned out—it was still going on when I left that agency—but I remember how the adversarial process haunted the defendants. I'm not sure how well I could do my job with that sort of judgment pending.

Should prices of medical procedures be required for informed consent? Perhaps. According to thefreedictionary.com, informed consent is "assent to permit an occurrence . . . that is based on a complete disclosure of facts needed to make the decision intelligently." I don't know if that's the best definition of informed consent, or even the correct legal one, but it's a good starting point for discussion.

To me, making an intelligent decision about health care often involves an awareness of the dollars involved. I'm not saying cost is the most important factor—just another consideration, like difficulty, discomfort, complications, recovery time, and likelihood of success.

Unlike most service providers, EMS agencies don't usually set prices according to supply and demand, because patients don't get to pick whose ambulance will respond to their 9-1-1 calls. Without competition, the biggest advantage to knowing prices up front is the opportunity to decline a particular intervention. Some would argue it's dangerous to give non-medical people that much discretion, but I think it would be possible to associate prices with brief, dummied-down summaries of recommended services. With a little cooperation from our employers, accessing such details wouldn't have to be any more complicated than looking up a medication on our smartphones.

The Lovely Helen agrees costs should be a bigger factor in health-care decisions. Like me, she doesn't understand why more patients don't ask us for prices. She also says the next time I'm sick, she's calling the vet.

Author's Note

Joey, our beloved Cav, died peacefully one evening soon after I wrote this. Now we have Charlie and Tiffany, two adorable dogs who think they're people.

DEATH
AFTER LIFE

2011

I had a pretty terrific childhood, thanks to my family and friends like Gary and Joel. We came of age during the '60s, when generations of civic values were challenged by social instability. That should have mattered more to us, but we were too busy testing limits imposed by parents, teachers, bosses, and bartenders.

Last autumn, Gary and I visited Joel at his home in Kansas. Joel had been sick. I didn't know much about his condition until I saw him for the first time in 37 years. Joel, whose size and physical prowess as a young man had been equal to Gary's plus mine, was gaunt and stooped, like so many cancer patients I'd seen. I felt myself sliding into medic mode despite my reluctance to turn our reunion into a house call.

I wasn't surprised when Joel died in May. I wasn't anything. According to my hard-wired Kennedy-era sensibilities, mourning was a luxury neither John Wayne nor I could afford. Both of us had to keep our heads clear to deal with the next indignity, or rescue, or Indian uprising. Death, to me, had become just another outcome, declared and documented whenever time, training, or technology wasn't enough.

I've written before about the dangers of red-bagging emotions. Lately, I've tried taking my own advice, so easily dispensed in the abstract: Feel, speak, heal. I'm omitting the part about which button to push to make that happen, possibly because I have no idea.

Since the American Heart Association literally wrote the book on critical care, I went back to my ACLS text for answers. The only guidance I could find about dealing with death is to accept pronouncement as the end of life. I'm fine with that—when I'm the one doing the pronouncing. It's different for families of the newly dead.

Psychiatrist Elizabeth Kübler-Ross wrote that grief often presents in five stages: denial, anger, bargaining, depression, and acceptance. I didn't sense any of those when Joel died. Maybe I wasn't supposed to. Kübler-Ross eventually downplayed her theory and conceded "There is not a typical response to loss, as there is no typical loss." I'd say Joel's death was "atypical" for me; he was a close friend, not a patient. Shouldn't that have made it easier to grieve?

Years of censoring sadness often leave us spiritually tongue-tied when facing tragedy away from our 9-1-1 world. It takes time for sentiments to spool up, even at a safe distance from EMS. Some of us never regain a desire to feel. That's a big sacrifice, just to stay numb to the random horrors of rescue. Stoicism looks good on tape but compromises health and home life when no one is watching.

Some colleagues present with reactionary feelings rather than repressed ones. To them, everything is funny and everything is sad. You'll find their punch lines about human frailty in the chat room of your choice. Take the high road with those folks; they're hurting, too.

EMS alters our death perception. Unlike the public, we react more to the dying than the dead. Our jobs require as much in the absence of advance directives or family decisions to the contrary. When patients die in our presence, that's as hard as it gets. I try retreating to a safe corner of my psyche to sidestep the emotional static of end-stage living, but that doesn't always work. I think most coworkers respond as I do, although Kübler-Ross says, "Our grieving is as individual as our lives." Perhaps that's true outside of EMS. There isn't much room for individuality in an industry driven by protocols and peer pressure.

The best approach for me has been to differentiate between death as an outcome and death as a loss. The former is unpleasant business; the latter is personal. It's taken me a long time to recognize a sense of loss as something to build on, rather than something to avoid.

I realized what I miss most when I lose someone close is the link between that person and my past. I began to visualize my life as a wheel with me at the hub, and spokes representing connections between people and memories. When death intrudes, spokes break and the wheel becomes wobbly. The only way to stabilize it is to replace old spokes with new ones; make fresh memories with friends and family. To dwell on broken spokes—connections that no longer exist—is to accentuate loss, rather than to accept it.

The patient-provider relationship in EMS shouldn't qualify for hub-spoke treatment. That doesn't mean we don't care about outcomes; we can be sympathetic and conscientious without vesting in memories. Sometimes, we even give families a little more time to prepare for their own grieving.

Thanks, Joel. I think I get it now.

References

Coping with grief and loss. http://www.helpguide.org/mental/grief loss.htm.

Henry, Mark C., and Edward R. Stapleton. *EMT Prehospital Care, Third Edition.* Mosby Jems, 2004.

HOW TO TELL A GOOD WAR STORY

2009

Last July, the National Association of State EMS Officials published a guide to help regional EMS systems compare local standards of care to national practices. After rereading the document, I realized there's a significant omission in the proposed curriculum: We don't teach our students how to tell war stories. As an aged but high-functioning member of the caregiving community, I consider it my duty to fill that void.

War stories are lurid, frequently embellished accounts of allegedly dangerous and/or heroic exploits, with the teller as protagonist. Their purpose is to impress, entertain, and most importantly, elicit nods and grunts of affirmation from a sympathetic crowd. According to a retrospective study of my memories—an alternative to time-consuming research—the ratio of nods to grunts is highest among small, EMS-only audiences, especially when the narrative includes words like "large-bore" and "cric."

Some would say war stories educate. Fair enough. Here's what I've learned from EMS war stories:

- Real medics can insert 14-gauge catheters into capillaries. In the dark. On horseback.
- If you knock on the wrong door and a deranged drug lord answers, your options are to hit him with your radio, fake a seizure, or pose as a stethoscope salesman.
- Bad calls are really good calls.

- The American Heart Association must have overlooked hundreds of saves from precordial thumps.
- You can intubate from more positions than there are in the *Kama Sutra*.
- Sometimes you have to do what you have to do. Sometimes you need a lawyer when you're done doing it.

Maybe war stories aren't all that illuminating. They have other uses, though. Suppose you're at a cocktail party and the talk turns to, say, the trade gap with Ghana. You'd be doing everyone a favor by rehashing your latest encounter with impaled body parts. By the time you finish, guests will admire you, feel sorry for you, or dread you.

War stories also are offered by some EMS instructors as substitutes for boring didactic material. Take pharmacology, for example. It's a lot easier for teachers and students to skip all that pedantic text about epinephrine dosing. Besides, when's the last time you gave epi for something as exciting as an evisceration?

The first thing you should know about war stories is that *what* happened isn't as important as *where*. Suppose I tell you I bagged, intubated, and resuscitated a patient; that's not nearly as impressive as claiming I bagged, intubated, and resuscitated that patient *while tethered to a fire escape!*

Next, war stories should convey a demure determination to do something dramatic, preferably against all odds. If the best you can do is describe how you helped an arthritic neighbor negotiate a child-resistant cap, you should probably keep that to yourself.

If you'd like to spin your very own war story, try the template below. Simply select from the multiple choices and you'll be the proud author of six sentences loaded with danger, decisiveness, perseverance, and poignancy.

1. **We responded to**
   - a train versus Ferris wheel.
   - a stand-off between cops and killer clowns.
   - an ice cream truck without exact change.
2. **I could see**
   - desolation where newly condemned warehouses once stood.
   - a cloud shaped like a eucalyptus tree.
   - clearly now, the rain is gone.

3. **I sensed that**
   - all my skills as an ACLS instructor would be needed.
   - all my skills as a game warden would be needed.
   - I should have taken that job at the post office.
4. **My first patient was**
   - Major General Hiram S. Dreedle of the Counter-MCI Task Force.
   - Skippy the Wonder Dog.
   - Gleck, from the planet Flurnoy.
5. **I knew I had to act fast, so I**
   - cranked open the O_2, then checked my e-mail.
   - said a little prayer to Azuza, goddess of the Transitional Layer.
   - called for my tube kit, but it didn't answer.
6. **It was touch and go, but I knew we'd made it when**
   - my relief arrived with fresh cravats.
   - I pushed the drug labeled "For really bad calls."
   - my patient got up and left.

I've always been reluctant to tell war stories. Maybe that's because I've found my most challenging cases in unexciting nursing homes. Managing elderly patients with acute illnesses, multiple meds, altered mental status, fragile vasculature, limited history, and concurrent, debilitating conditions won't make the evening news. Besides, what self-respecting medic would start a war story with, "There I was at the senior center . . . ?"

I'm going to have to start hanging out downtown. With my tube kit.

LEGACY IN THE DUST

2011

The last time 9/11 was known only as the day after 9/10, Larry Zacarese was sleeping in. "I'd been working plain clothes in Jamaica [NY]," the 35-year-old police officer and paramedic remembers, "and was supposed to start my vacation that morning. Instead, I got a call from my mother about planes crashing into buildings."

Larry drove very fast to his precinct, the 113th, then continued toward the nearest bridge linking Long Island to the target-rich environment known as Manhattan. His trek was interrupted by an unrelated shooting. The victim, who needed a priest more than a cop or a medic, would be Larry's only patient that day.

Zacarese reached Ground Zero mid-afternoon, joined by like-minded responders whose life-saving skills were limited to scenarios not involving ballistic airliners. He spent the next three days doing 12-hour shifts—for 14-15 hours. "I told my dad, 'I'm not coming home until I find somebody.' I was convinced we'd pull people out. I just wanted to get one person out."

Days became weeks, then months. By December, Larry's tour of duty at the country's biggest crime scene had tapered to one or two days a week. It was time to return to Jamaica, but not for long. In March, Zacarese achieved a long-term goal by joining NYPD's elite Emergency Services Unit (ESU). There he met Captain Barry Galfano, who would become his mentor and friend. Like Larry, Galfano had worked at Ground Zero almost every day until December. Then, with no one to rescue, Galfano had dedicated himself to supporting the living. "[As a Captain] I had the ability to go up to people and say, 'I know you're hurting. We're all hurting. We've got to pull through,' Galfano said. "That became one of my biggest functions down there."

★★★

Larry was almost through ESU's four-month training when he was diagnosed with reactive airway disease and a site-specific malady known as World Trade Center (WTC) cough. Unable to achieve a peak flow suitable for ESU's scuba mission, the third-generation NYPD veteran knew he'd have to choose a different assignment. Galfano, who'd commanded a K-9 unit earlier in his career, convinced his protégé to follow that route. It wasn't easy, but Zacarese got through it in 16 weeks. "K-9 was the toughest training I did," Larry confides. "By then, I was using an inhaler to help me catch my breath."

Zacarese is one of approximately 6,000 adults exposed to WTC debris who suffered new-onset asthma. Some estimates put that number twice as high. Workers who arrived at Ground Zero on 9/11 and spent at least three months on the pile have shown the highest rate of respiratory illness. Forced expiratory volume, a measure of lung function, remains well below normal for more than 10% of the firefighters, cops, and EMS workers who were part of the recovery effort.

Those folks had more than a casual knowledge of hazmat. Weren't they worried about ongoing exposure to vaporized skyscrapers?

For Galfano, an environmental science background helped make the consequences of his duty pretty clear. "I knew I was breathing smoke and chemicals," he said, "and I'm telling myself, 'Twenty years from now you're going to end up with lung cancer,' but we still had a job to do. We still had to recover bodies, recover all our people."

★★★

By 2004, Zacarese was feeling more winded. He developed a persistent rash and added GERD and sleep apnea to his job-related illnesses. His list of medications started to resemble a formulary for COPDers twice his age. "I was tired all the time. It became a quality-of-life issue."

In June of 2009, two years after being promoted to Sergeant, Larry left NYPD to become assistant chief of police and director of emergency management at Stony Brook University. He also attends law school and works as a paramedic in Suffolk County. He knows he's lucky to be as healthy as a 60-year-old two-pack-a-day smoker. "A lot of guys are much worse off," he concedes.

Galfano, whom many subordinates credit with helping them through the horrors of 9/11, underwent surgery in 2008 for a malignant tumor in his small intestine. Within two years, cancer had spread to his legs, lungs, liver, and brain. He died while I was writing this.

Barry Galfano and Larry Zacarese represent thousands of emergency services workers for whom rescue and leadership—not scene safety and back-up—were the first priorities on 9/11. Our textbooks were right: You can get hurt that way. What the textbooks don't teach is that no one should be left behind. I'm proud to know people who get that.

Author's Note

Zacarese added attorney to his other occupations and ran for Suffolk County sheriff in 2017. He says he misses Galfano every day.

ANAL MEDICS
Don't Be A-Freud

2011

In college, I had a Contemporary Civilization professor who fancied himself a Freudian. This was in the early '70s, when it was still fashionable to do so. As an engineering student trying to maintain consciousness during an interminable psych lecture, I probably wasn't paying much attention—until my instructor addressed anal retentiveness. He might as well have been profiling me.

Freud theorized that infants progress from oral to anal stages characterized by obsession with bowel control. As I recall (I must have stayed awake for some of that class), anal retentive children wait until they're maxed-out on encouragement before letting nature take over. I may have acted that way as a one-year-old. I don't remember—I was very young at the time. What I do know is I have traits considered anal by family, friends, and even editors.

I think being anal makes me a better caregiver. I'm determined to convince the rest of you that anal medics, though we may be mocked, have a purpose in EMS no less consequential than any combination of airway, breathing, and circulation you favor.

My dictionary defines anal behavior as "orderly, stingy, stubborn, etc." No doubt "etc" was inserted by some lazy writer with anal envy. I'll come back to that.

I think I've outgrown stingy; no longer do I deny friends postage stamps, as I did in school because "they're mine." As for stubborn, some might claim I'm not, but only if they're confusing me with someone else. That leaves orderly. Guilty as charged. I crave order. I'll fight for order. If you're between me and order, you're going down—well, only if I can do that without getting messy. (When you're anal, neatness counts.)

Order is a good thing in EMS. Order begins even before you report to work. Order means someone you'll relieve has checked supplies and equipment on your ambulance, has removed patient detritus and restocked whatever's missing, has finished the shift's paperwork, and left the ready room neat, if not pristine. It's not fair for all that work to be delegated to one person, but that's a cross anal-ytics often bear without complaint—assuming our noble efforts to remediate others don't count as complaints.

I used to work with a world-class anal medic. Let's call him Al (guess if you must, but that's not even close to his real name). Al's co-workers considered him quirky and a bit of a nuisance. He'd find expired angiocaths before anyone else knew plastic had a half-life. He'd empty sharps containers while there was still room at the top. He'd check BP cuffs for off-center gauges. When you rode with Al, you knew you had enough of everything—2×2's, 3×3's, 2.3×3.2s—to handle at least a dozen calls without resupplying. Al's bosses and partners made fun of him, but when Al was off, there was a preparation gap that occasionally deprived Al's colleagues of very useful items—electrodes or charged batteries, for example. During after-hours titration of liquid refreshment, everyone agreed Al was indispensable . . . and a pain in the butt.

I think we need more Als in EMS, which is why I'd like to go back to that dictionary definition of anal and replace "etc" with "organized, conscientious, and thorough." (Is it too late to add humble?) To earn those adjectives, I offer this occupational checklist. I call it Six Degrees of Preparation:

√ **Personal equipment.** Is my uniform clean? Do I have my stuff (whatever I normally carry)? Does it work?
√ **Company equipment.** Is my vehicle stocked? Will it start? Does it need fuel, fluid, or air? Are there any issues with medical equipment? Are batteries charged?
√ **Continuing education.** How's my recertification progressing? Do I need to register for upcoming classes or exams?
√ **Health.** Am I well enough to work safely and effectively?
√ **Attitude.** Do I still care enough to treat patients the way I'd like to be treated, regardless of presenting problem, demographics, or proximity to the end of my shift?

√   **Outside issues.** Will personal problems distort my focus, putting me, my partner, or my patients at risk?

Being anal doesn't mean obsessing over these items. It's more about enforcing one's own good habits. Those of you lacking the anal gene can play, too. Go ahead—we're not contagious.

Freud may have been an alarmist about toilet training, but I think his prudent appraisal of anal personalities can promote understanding and appreciation of detail-oriented people in EMS. We're obligate risk managers. We're success driven. We value quality over quantity. We're reliable.

Besides, who else is going to count all those 4×4s?

CULTURE CLUB

2013

A long time ago at an agency far, far away, someone smarter than I am said I needed a life outside of EMS. That astute observation was probably based on my habit of commuting directly between my paying EMS job and my volunteer agency. I did that mostly because I was attracted to the customs, skills, and opinions of paid and unpaid people with whom I served. Our shared practices were, to me, the essence of rescue. Some would call it culture. My question is, does EMS have one?

Firefighters do. I know that because they tell me so. More than one has pinpointed their near-palpable culture as the biggest difference between them and us. I believe that, but I also think cultural gaps between fire and EMS are less about what we do and more about how long we've been doing it. Compared to fire, EMS is just getting started.

I once asked a firefighter who was also a paramedic to name all aspects of fire culture that came to mind. He mentioned danger, physicality, worth, camaraderie, and discipline. I have no basis to argue with any of that. I've never been a firefighter and it's not on my bucket list. At 60, I'm quite sure a try-out in turnout gear would teach me more about geriatrics than firematics. When I consider my colleague's summation of fire's culture from an EMS perspective, though, I think we measure up pretty well:

Danger

As a child in the 1950s, I was aware of three fundamental threats: sharp objects, busy streets, and fire. I figured people who engaged the latter to protect the rest of us were very brave. I've never doubted that or the dangers of firefighting. However, now that I know more about disease, disability, and how hopelessly deranged some patients and bystanders are, I feel EMS is just as risky.

Physicality

I used to think physical demands separated firefighting from other essential services. That was before I spent 20 years carrying patients, equipment, and patients with equipment. A few weeks in EMS were enough to acquaint me with muscles I didn't know I had. During that first year, I started to see definition in my limbs that I hadn't noticed since I'd retired from competitive hockey. I'm not saying I was ever strong enough to carry a 200-pounder safely down a ladder, but hauling even 50 pounds hundreds of feet three or four times a day definitely gets the blood flowing.

Worth

It's hard to gauge the value to society of EMS or any essential service. Even labeling EMS *essential* is presumptuous, although I don't think most people who call us would argue with that classification.

In business, value is usually determined by what a willing buyer pays a willing seller, but that assumption is less accurate when customers purchase services from monopolies like our local 9-1-1 systems. To me, fire and EMS seem equally capable of meeting urgent, narrowly scoped needs.

Camaraderie

Firefighting is usually much more of a group activity than prehospital care is. I'm sure teamwork promotes unity within a firehouse; however, I don't think there's a closer, non-familial relationship than what many pairs of EMS partners share.

Discipline

Let's consider two kinds of discipline: internal and external.

Internal discipline is about projecting and respecting authority. Having worked for both fire and EMS organizations, I'd say this is no contest. Compliance with boundaries and responsibilities mediated by chains of command seems much higher in the fire service.

External discipline is the extent to which we obey other people's rules. I think firefighters and EMS providers are similarly predisposed: We improvise, we adapt, we overcome, and we have little patience with anyone who interferes with that process.

Culture is evolutionary—not manufactured nor awarded. Nascent EMS traditions like those above must mix and meld to make an institution greater than the sum of its parts. Consider Scotch, aged in barrels before being sold; the ingredients have been there since day one, but maturation takes time. Rushing that process is beyond the bounds of human endeavor.

Firefighters can boast of a culture because the fire service has existed for more than 300 years. We can admire fire's rich history, but we gain little by comparing ourselves to them. They've earned what they have, and so will we someday.

Let's not be in a hurry to claim our culture. Like whiskey, EMS will improve with age.

PERFORMANCE ANXIETY

2014

Once in a while, I do a little acting. I mean besides feigning exhaustion when it's time to wash the dishes. I'm talking about short, educational skits in front of fellow EMS providers, where I play a paramedic working in nontraditional settings. I can always count on my Opryland connections for fresh material about show business medicine, and for a limitless supply of very talented cast members who, unlike me, can actually sing and dance.

While rehearsing our routines, I was struck by the similarities between EMS and entertainment.

Professionals in both disciplines appreciate the value of practice and the need to get it before doing it for real. There's respect for experience without discounting the possibility a newcomer might contribute something of value. When the unexpected occurs—an extra patient, for example, or a broken mic—partners/performers adapt promptly and wordlessly, usually without patients or audience members aware of improvisation.

Like singers who begin by studying breath control, EMS professionals learn the science of patient care before exploring the art. Supplementary business and communication classes make paramedics more marketable in much the same way voice and ballet lessons enhance actors' versatility. Attributes of accomplished entertainers—timing, personality, self-control—match up well with desirable traits of caregivers.

That's as far as the parallels go for me.

Acting is just for fun, without life-and-death consequences for missed cues. I'm comfortable on stage because I'm accustomed to working in front of people. As a real medic treating real patients, however, I'm uneasy about being watched.

I know my performances won't be dissected to the same extent actors are reviewed by critics, but part of me realizes even subtle aspects of my behavior contribute to bystanders' impressions of me and my profession. Even when I make good decisions, some of what I do in the field—temporarily ignoring traumatized extremities to treat critical conditions, for example—doesn't necessarily look correct to untrained observers. Such misunderstandings can lead to second-guessing, sometimes extended by word of mouth to people who weren't even on scene. Concern about such possibilities shouldn't ever interfere with patient care, but having to manage perception-vs.-reality gaps is fatiguing and can certainly up our anxiety quotients.

I'm reminded of a cardiac arrest I treated while I was the sole EMS provider on duty at a concert a few years ago. The elderly male had been down less than a minute when someone summoned me to his side. He was in v-fib. I called for manpower, showed an onlooker how to do chest compressions, defibrillated, and was inserting an OPA when the patient woke up in a sinus rhythm and wanted to know what happened.

Pretty much a best-case scenario, wouldn't you say? Not according to a colleague, who passed along a rumor that the arrest hadn't been managed properly. I can only guess someone in the crowd thought resuscitation doesn't count unless compressions are accompanied by ventilations. Then there was the comment from Security that I hadn't adequately communicated the urgency of the situation. I guess that explains why they didn't show up.

Any branch of a prehospital decision tree might determine a call's outcome. That's a big enough burden for responders. When patient care becomes a spectacle, though, as it sometimes does when illness or injury strikes in a crowded venue, rescuers have to work even harder to optimize results. Developing "stage presence" can help.

To me, stage presence is a combination of attitude and aptitude. It tells your audience you've done this before, you enjoy it, and you're good at it. At its simplest level in EMS, stage presence is about managing a scene as effortlessly as possible. Making a big production of patient care gets noticed, but is no more desirable than drowning out the lyrics of a gentle ballad with dance-club clatter.

What kinds of prehospital practices enhance stage presence?

- Maintaining eye contact with patients while assessing their mental status, circulation, and respiratory effort
- Allowing clarification—not interference—from bystanders
- Verbalizing treatment and transport recommendations calmly yet persuasively
- Proceeding purposefully with time-sensitive therapeutics

All contribute to a perception of proficient caregivers as experienced, confident, and in control. Crowds are less likely to become distractions, I think, when on-scene proceedings seem scripted to spectators. Like gifted entertainers, the best among us make it all look easy.

FROM A DISTANCE

2014

A year ago, I left my last clinical position in EMS. My back had started to demand more of my attention than patients on some calls. I decided to walk away while I still could—a state my gimpy left leg reminds me I shouldn't take for granted.

I'm not done with EMS; I still read about it, write about it, even dream about it. I also miss it, a lot . . . well, not all of it. Working in snow, for example. I hate snow. I'm glad I don't have to respond when it's snowing, or when it's cold enough to snow, or when people say it might snow. We get tornadoes and other wrath-of-God storms every few weeks in Tennessee, but at least it doesn't snow much.

Here are some things about EMS I don't miss, besides snow:

Harsh tones from telephones, pagers, and radios. I still flinch when the phone rings. I've read it has something to do with a heightened startle reflex. Good thing I don't do IVs anymore. Or serve the soup course.

Meaningless administrative practices. I didn't mind a little paperwork, but documenting obscure demographics was particularly irritating. I'm waiting for research that correlates patients' outcomes to their occupations.

The absurdity of treating the sick while sick. When I was in the corporate world, we were expected to work even when we were germ-ridden. That would be ridiculous on so many levels in EMS, wouldn't it? Anyone?

Unstable respiratory patients. Watching someone struggle to breathe is especially hard, I think, because we've all been short of breath. Ninth-inning Red Sox rallies still do that to me.

The real meaning of HIPAA. "How I Prevent Administrative Action," I'd guess, referencing data gatekeepers who arbitrarily and unnecessarily invoke HIPAA as a barrier to clinical QA/QI. There are legitimate, unobtrusive ways of giving EMS providers objective feedback about patient outcomes.

Parents who don't advocate for their kids. I was amazed at the risks some parents took on behalf of their children. Moms and dads whose pursuit of entertainment was interrupted by sick or injured kids often tried negotiating with me to delay definitive care. The worst part was knowing even clueless parents have the final say.

Maternity calls. What scared me about birthing babies was all that stuff I've never done but would have had to do if something other than a head presented. Practicing with a plastic perineum was pretty far from reassuring.

Different protocols in different regions for the same diseases, same species. It's like having different rules for baseball east and west of the Mississippi.

Most of my EMS memories are pleasant, though:

Good calls with good outcomes. Seeing patients wake up after treatment made me wonder why I'd waited so long to get into EMS.

The value of paying attention in class. I loved discovering, *Hey, that actually works!* the first time I'd try something theoretical on a real patient.

Partners with good advice. Nothing against wives, but sometimes you need a friend who doesn't know you *that* well.

Partners with good ideas. I can't count the times my coworkers knew a better way and made it so.

Learning, trying, teaching. I'm not sure there's any such thing as an observer in EMS. Whatever orientation time I thought I had, or was told I had, was always overestimated. Maybe that doesn't sound like a positive, but I usually preferred doing to watching. Soon after doing came teaching, which I still think is the best way to learn.

Sharing a noble profession with like-minded people. There's a sweet spot within an us-against-the-world mentality where you celebrate, rather than resent, what makes you different.

Being needed. My daughter needed me and my wife still needs me (at times), but being needed by total strangers made going to work seem worthwhile even when I wasn't at my best.

I think I've adjusted fairly well to life without protocols. I look forward to most days, even without that surge of anticipation I used to feel on my way to calls. I'd like a little more money in the bank—who wouldn't?—but not if it meant working in offices the past 22 years.

I've learned more about the human condition than any fellow engineer I know. I've been to the brink and back; it's time to move on. Or maybe I could still do per diem . . .

Author's Note

There are two occupations I still have magical thoughts about pursuing: ice hockey and EMS. Those are equally ridiculous goals, given my age and physical condition.

I threw out all my hockey stuff so I wouldn't be tempted to join a senior league, but I still have my stethoscope and an old pair of work boots. And maybe a pair of BDUs. And a jacket with patches. Hmm . . .

SOCIALIZED MEDICINE

2014

When I accepted a paramedic position at Opryland seven years ago, my Human Resources contact said she recommended me for the job not because of my experience, references, clean record, or willingness to dress like a grown-up. She liked me because I smiled a lot.

I was surprised to hear that. Smiling isn't a natural act for me. When I smile, it's usually forced and comes across as a grimace or sneer. There are worse problems to have, but it bothers me to think of the many budding acquaintances I may have inadvertently sabotaged because I couldn't coordinate the muscles of my face. I was lucky Opryland interviewed me on a day when my mouth was synchronized with the rest of me.

Smiling is a higher priority at Opryland than at other EMS venues because the primary business is relaxation, not medicine. Albert Schweitzer wouldn't last at Opryland if he couldn't direct hotel patrons to the swimming pool with a smile. EMS is just another aspect of customer service when your patients are also your guests.

At first, I thought Opryland's emphasis on pleasantries might infringe on medical matters. It's hard to chat about recreation with fun-seekers when you're sticking needles into them. By the end of my first year, though, I started to appreciate an EMS/entertainment hybrid—the social medic—whose amiability and maturity are at least as important as clinical competence.

You don't have to be a paramedic to be a social medic at Opryland. "Medic" means any employee with EMS certification. Responders don't wear patches; the emphasis is on service, not certification. All workers, including EMS personnel, are considered equally qualified to help guests enjoy their stay. When a patient feels good about an experience with an Opryland medic, it's probably because the interaction complemented, rather than disrupted, the guest's vacation.

It's not unusual for EMTs and paramedics who work outside of 9-1-1 systems to be considered minor leaguers by their street-centric peers. I know that because I felt that way, and so did most of my partners when I was in the field. Now that I've done both, I realize the social skills of practitioners at non-traditional EMS sites are often underrated. Consider, for example, these desirable characteristics of caregivers at entertainment venues:

Good communicator. You might be able to substitute professional detachment for rapport with emergent patients, but the majority of cases in a recreational environment require little more than pleasant conversation. Empathetic, congenial words spoken effortlessly foster a can-do image that facilitates problem solving.

Likes people. When folks pay to stay with you, they expect a respite from the petty indignities of life without room service. If you don't enjoy the company of humans, you'll likely project ambivalence about your job that might remind guests why they needed a vacation.

Not a diva. I'm using that term figuratively to describe medics of both genders who opt for the dramatic when the therapeutic will do. We all know people like that. Working in entertainment doesn't mean you're star of the show.

Slow to anger. You've just Heimliched a diner's last bite of brisket into orbit and are feeling pretty good about your standing in the universe, when your patient's spouse asks if they're going to be charged for the meal. As imperative as it might seem to deliver a lecture on priorities, any reply other than a polite answer to the billing question would be inappropriate.

Good "bench" skills. There won't be time to Google how to sling and swathe a shoulder injury when your impatient patient is late for a show. If your basic repertoire is rusty, consider spending more time in the company of manikins.

Part entertainer, part educator. Entertainment is about adding value to customers' expectations. You don't have to be P. T. Barnum to do that. Taking extra time with patients to explain findings and options almost guarantees you won't be considered a weak link in your company's service.

I don't think there's a single trait in the above list you wouldn't want your street medics to have, too.

The social medic isn't an aberration, but rather a progression of caregiving skills from clinical to comprehensive. With community paramedicine on the horizon, EMS providers will have to offer more than dispassionate emergent care. Personality, patience, and a willingness to commit to something less than lifesaving are attributes worth exhibiting the next time you look for a job.

Smiling wouldn't hurt, either.

NO MEAT LOAF
FOR LUCY

2012

I am married to a world-class cook. I'd be grateful for that even if I weren't in EMS. My own, stunted capabilities in the kitchen leave me at the mercy of anyone who knows the difference between poached and parboiled.

Shifts punctuated by chow more convenient than nutritious make sit-down meals with the family special. I enjoy feasting as I imagine our forefathers did—after our fore*mothers* picked, plucked, skinned, scaled, or otherwise rendered edible the day's protein. Hearty fare like a roast or a stew has that homespun feel that still resonates, I think, with most of us in Marcus Welby's target audience. Besides, eating at home is a lot safer than ingesting food-like substances of questionable pedigree between transports—a high-stakes game I call The Good, The Bad, and The Cholinergic.

It's not that all street food is dangerous—just unpredictable. A dairy-derived entrée ordered on a hot summer day from the most fastidious, color-coordinated franchise can cause more distress than a burrito from a body-shop vending machine. Stress is also a factor; that side order of catecholamines is a recipe for dyspepsia. And trying to time meal breaks with the ebb and flow of the rescue business is about as frustrating as forecasting the stock market.

Like wilderness medicine or high-angle rescue, selection of mid-shift nourishment is a sub-specialty of EMS. There are many variables; you have to minimize cost and square footage of edibles while optimizing speed of delivery (quality is desirable but improbable). Success is defined by The Rule of Fives: food in five minutes for less than five dollars, requiring no more than five fingers to eat. Doing that math while navigating a drive-up window is an acquired skill—like kneeling near but not in body fluids. Yes, there are reasons why street grub makes me think of body fluids.

It's no exaggeration to portray chow as central to the ethos of EMS:

- In Martin Scorsese's *Bringing Out the Dead*, suicidal paramedic Frank Pierce's partner, Larry (played by John Goodman), takes pride in planning the perfect overnight take-out hours in advance.
- Medics rush from a taco stand to their next call in 1998's disturbing *Broken Vessels*.
- Kathy Bates stars as food critic and EMT Jane Stern in *Ambulance Girl*.

An aspect of rescue not commonly publicized during primary training is the right to declare a food emergency if partners cannot agree on cuisine. During food emergencies, it is customary for the senior medic to dictate a mealtime destination—unless a much larger junior crew member raised by wolves starts using words like "gnaw" and "eviscerate."

Store-bought food in the field feels emergent. Like patients, I have a right to refuse AMA—Awesome Meal Awaits—whenever Helen has something cooking at home. It's hard to overrate her definitive care for acute hunger. That's not the only reason I married her, but it's definitely in the top 10.

I can't claim The Lovely Helen's kitchen prowess is unanimously appreciated in our household. I'm pretty sure our Cavalier King Charles spaniel, Lucy, wishes my wife were a wiz at, say, landscaping instead. Then there might be leftover human snacks to augment Lucy's diet of kibbles and nibbles, or whatever they call Cheerios for dogs.

Last week, for example, Helen made her to-die-for meat loaf. I know, "meat loaf" sounds uninspired, but we're talking savory, succulent slices of ground beef, pork, and veal, wrapped in bacon and bathed in brown gravy. Grown men weep in anticipation. Vegans ask for seconds. I was well into thirds when I heard Helen tell Lucy to be patient, there was a piece for her. Yes, Helen speaks Spaniel.

"Not so fast," I said, or something equally charitable. I knew Helen's meat loaf was much tastier and healthier than anything I'd consider consuming at work. I was already planning portions that would optimize the size and number of meals I could bring from home. Lucy's ration, I'm ashamed to admit, became her donation to my campaign against hunger in EMS.

I sympathize, Lucy. Our DNA is so similar, if the weather had been a few degrees cooler 50 million years ago I'd be begging for your bone.

Author's Note

Ah, Lucy—Cav #3. She lived another year or so until her kidneys gave out. Pets steal your heart like you thought only your kids could.

MD ENVY

2009

Here's a question for my paramedic brethren: Did anyone ever have to remind you you're not a doctor? Your partner, perhaps? Your boss? A judge?

A Korean War corpsman nearing retirement delivered that message to me during my first year of practice. I had just delayed our departure from the local ER by reciting obscure differentials, scavenged from memories of multiple-choice exams, to my patient's bemused physician.

"You know," my partner said, "you ought to change that 'EMT-P' after your name to 'AAD.'"

"What's AAD?" I asked.

"Almost A Doctor."

Got it.

My colleague had correctly diagnosed me with MD Envy, a humiliating but treatable condition presenting with any of the following signs:

- You carry more prehospital meds in your car than the neighborhood pharmacy stocks.
- You favor physician oversight—for other medics.
- Your diagnoses correlate to last week's *House* reruns.
- You think the only difference between you and a doctor is $150K a year.
- You spend hours on the Internet searching for paramedic-to-physician bridge programs.

I'm not sure why we sometimes think we're smarter than doctors. Maybe we confuse skills with knowledge. Sure, we might have more recent experience inserting airways and IVs than, say, the dermatologist who just cut that mole off your back, but that doesn't mean our curriculum approaches the depth and detail of a physician's. Perhaps it's unrealistic to expect us to grasp the exponential differences in training and accountability between our two disciplines.

I remember a lunchtime discussion with an ED attending and several EMS coworkers about a paramedic who'd attempted a pre-hospital C-section to save the fetus of a mortally injured mother. The sentiment around the table was mostly supportive of the medic's actions. Only the physician dissented. His point was, "You'd have to be a doctor to know why you'd have to be a doctor" to safely perform such an advanced procedure. I agree it's difficult to make good decisions with only superficial knowledge of pros and cons.

Even interventions within our scope of practice can be risky without recent experience. For example, I worked in a system with a prehospital protocol specifying repeated intubation and extubation to suction aspirated meconium. If I count the neonatal intubations I've done in the field, add them to the number of meconium births I've witnessed, then multiply by two just to impress you, I still get zero. Sometimes we have to stretch our comfort zone, but it's dangerous to substitute willingness for competence.

I think much of our self-image as AADs is wishful thinking spurred by our earliest prehospital successes. Favorable short-term outcomes after treating manageable but incurable conditions like diabetes and asthma can distort our perception of EMS's limitations and leave us feeling omnipotent. With enough positive reinforcement from patients and peers, some of us begin to view higher education as an option, rather than a prerequisite for entry into the gated community of professional healers.

Another cause of MD envy is Hollywood's progressive portrayal of physicians as more vulnerable and less stoic than their predecessors (think Mark Greene vs. Ben Casey). It's easier for us to identify with doctors who are sleep-deprived and fallible than with the imperturbable, white-coated icons of my youth. The danger is allowing collegiality to inflate our sense of our own capabilities. Instead of thinking, *I've done easier procedures; therefore, I can do harder ones*, our oath to do no harm should discourage experimentation with risky treatment modalities suggested not by sound medicine, but by ambition.

Patients can potentiate pangs of MD envy, too. As a semi-unretired paramedic in the entertainment business, I treat many people who don't want to waste even an hour of their recreational time at a medical facility. I'd like to help them by reading X-rays and writing prescriptions, but I'm about seven years short on training. Consequently, there are sore throats, upset stomachs, swollen ankles, and twisted knees that never get definitive care. The best I can do is spot emergent issues, treat what I can, then lobby for transport to an ED. When my patients hear me say, "I'm a paramedic, not a doctor," as I try to avoid yet another refusal, some think it's just a posterior-protecting ploy. Mostly, it's an acknowledgment that my expertise is limited and I don't always know what I don't know.

For those of you whose MD envy is refractory to my well-intentioned guidance, there is a solution: Become a doctor. Or a nurse practitioner or a physician assistant. Each practice at much higher levels than the most gifted paramedics.

On the other hand, there's no shame in *not* being a doctor. If it were easy, I would have done it three decades ago just to pursue a childhood fascination with all things medical. Instead, I've adapted to my limitations and cultivated pride in EMS. I'd like to think there are plenty of people out there who envy *us*.

THE NARCAN
MONOLOGUES

2016

Those of you who are new to EMS . . . May I speak with you a minute?

You may have heard about this February Facebook post by a Weymouth, Massachusetts firefighter:

"Narcan is the worst drug ever created, let the scum bags die . . . I for one get no extra money for giving narcan (sic) and these losers are out of the hospital and using again in hours, you use you should loose (sic)!"

I'm wondering how you feel about that. I suppose it depends partly on whom you work with.

When I was a new medic, I couldn't help being swayed by the opinions of senior coworkers. They'd been living the life I wanted—working insane hours on the streets of New York City, racing each other to barely controlled scenes, packaging and transporting victims of every imaginable anatomical insult within minutes of arriving, toweling off sweat and blood, then lining up to do it again. I either idolized them or was afraid of them, so when they preached their gospel of empathy-free zones, I bought into it.

That doesn't mean we were right. I didn't know it at the time, but some of the ways my partners had adapted to working long hours in a frenetic 9-1-1 system weren't healthy. The cynicism I sensed from them—right around the time I started feeling it myself—triggers a distorted view of people, healthcare, and life in general. You tend to forget whatever attracted you to EMS in the first place. It's different for each provider, but I'm pretty sure none of us think we're ever going to hope patients die.

Part of me feels badly for that Weymouth firefighter. I can imagine him as one of my transports: a man whose glass is neither half empty nor half full, but rather overflowing with misery brought on by bad choices and flawed coping. "He's truly sorry," according to his chief. I'm not sure that matters.

If you want to do more than take up space in an ambulance, you'll have to find ways to be better than most of the folks you meet. I can't tell you how to do that, but I think it helps to gauge your sensibilities against the great mass of certified paramedical people once in a while. When you notice yourself automatically agreeing with the prevailing sentiments about scumbags, it's probably time to take a sick day and drain some of those hostilities. Reflect a bit on why EMS is worth doing.

You could start by reading the comments from your colleagues following that Weymouth Facebook post. I can pretty much promise you'll agree with only about half of them. The question is, which half? The one that thinks the firefighter must be having a bad day; that he has a right to his opinions, and we all secretly feel the same way?

I hope not.

You don't get to judge whether someone deserves your care. Not ever. And if you speak out publicly about the undesirability of certain patients—heroin addicts, for example—neither Facebook nor the First Amendment is going to protect you from being disciplined or even fired.

There is no number of years after which you earn the right to make sociopathic remarks. If you can't understand that, try looking at it from your employer's point of view: Would you take responsibility for someone whose goal in life is thinning the herd?

Making less money than the person you least admire doesn't justify mistreating people. As Weymouth's mayor Bob Hedlund said of the infamous post, "There are certain boundaries and responsibilities that come with the (EMS) job." Letting patients die when you have the means to save them is pretty far outside those boundaries. If there's a chance your feelings about Narcan, drugs, system abuses, or the color purple might cause you to withhold your region's standard of care, you can save yourself, your family, your partners, your employers, and at least a few hundred innocent citizens some very difficult times by engaging in an occupation that doesn't require human contact.

Those aren't my rules; they were here when I started in EMS. I'm just passing them along to you in case you work with people who are just as toasty as I was ten years ago. I had to relearn a lot about empathy while taking a year off.

Perhaps some of your partners should do the same.

Author's Note

Opiate abuse is still a national crisis and an excuse for EMS providers to publish their ugliest thoughts.

I PROTEST

2012

A few months ago, I spotted a question about fentanyl availability on a popular web site. Although we don't carry fentanyl
where I work, I was hoping to learn more about supplies of other
meds. Instead, I saw this comment about drug shortages: "Thank the
Obama administration for this. This is part of the culture of death being pushed by liberals."

Such rhetoric without rationale reminded me of 1972, an uneasy
time on the campus of Columbia University. I was a 19-year-old engineering student trying to maintain a 2.8 grade-point average while
steering clear of Vietnam-era conflict. Mostly, though, I was majoring
in meeting women, which is why I joined a rowdy, upper-Manhattan
march to protest something or other.

At Broadway and 96th Street, someone threw a rock at a bank.
Then someone else did the same. Pretty soon, stones flew from all
directions, aimed at stately, etched glass windows and police officers
standing in front of them. Some of the cops started running toward
us with batons raised. Having been absent from class the day they
covered guilt by association, I didn't retreat—well, not right away. I
waited until I saw the reds of the officers' eyes, then sprinted over—
not around—people, bushes, bicycles, traffic barriers, and at least one
NYPD cruiser. That was the end of my first and last protest march.

I felt fortunate to have avoided both incarceration and a gratuitous craniotomy. I also was relieved not to have had to explain to
parents or professors why I'd risked so much for a cause I couldn't
even name, much less justify. It had been so easy to simply go along
with others without asking why. We were too busy parroting the
slogans of the day: "Kill the pigs," "Right on, bomb Saigon," and the
ever popular "Ho, Ho, Ho Chi Minh, the NLF is going to win." We
felt superior to those who didn't get it, whatever "it" was. We didn't

understand that arbitrary acts and incendiary words often trample more rights than they protect.

I was curious about the person who posted that not-so-conservative remark about liberals, so I looked him up. He's a first responder, firefighter, and business owner. Now that I know that, there are two things I can tell you: I wouldn't do business with him and I wouldn't want him to respond to my emergency. Why would I put my property or my life in the hands of anyone who dismisses such a large portion of the population he's supposed to protect? Even if I'm not part of that segment, blatantly unsupportable generalizations reveal character flaws I'd rather not subsidize. It's possible to advocate, debate, and disagree without impulsively labeling opponents inferior or, even worse, dangerous. Civilization depends on such tolerance.

These are tough times for fire and EMS. Talk to those who walk in both worlds; they'll tell you public respect and resources have eroded since 9/11. Yes, we need to change, but some of that must originate from within. I'd like to see more thoughtful discourse, even when we assume such dialogue is strictly internal. We could certainly use the practice. Along the way, we'd learn to favor compromise and defuse rancor. Perhaps we could use those skills to market ourselves a little more effectively.

Back in the '70s, my classmates and I didn't blame liberals for the ills of the planet; we targeted bankers, senators, republicans, soldiers, astronauts, anyone over 40 (or was it 35?), cops, evangelists, rich white people, men with short hair, and poor old Dr. McGill—a nice man who happened to be president of my school for a few difficult years. We were too sanctimonious to recognize that we were guilty of the same arrogance we were protesting. We shorted progress for headlines and hate.

I see change as an iterative process, sparked but not driven by dissent. Whether the target is occupational or political, regional or national, the chances of success improve when advocates offer more than exaggeration and intimidation. Know the issues, set realistic goals, and above all, avoid hypocrisy.

As a witness to Chicago's 1969 "Days of Rage" riot yelled to demonstrators, "I don't know what your cause is, but you just set it back 100 years."

Author's Note

The trend toward uncompromising, adversarial stances via social media hasn't slowed in the nine years since I wrote this column. I'm not sure if it's an aberration or the new normal.

HEAD OF THE CLASS

2015

Teaching is not a lost art, but the regard for it is a lost tradition.

—Jacques Barzun, author and educator.

After giving and taking ACLS and PALS classes for 20 years, I generally expect less of those courses when I attend them past the midpoint of five-year AHA cycles. It's hard for teachers and students to get excited about covering the same material as last time.

That's why I was pleasantly surprised by my PALS instructor's engaging approach during a recent refresher. Elizabeth Clinard, RN—an ED nurse most days—annotated the compulsory videos with real-world commentary and was particularly good with first-time PALS students who needed lots of encouragement during practical exercises. At the end of the two-day session, the class's performance in the dreaded megacodes was the best I've seen.

Clinard must have understood that good teachers subordinate themselves to their material. If you think it's easy for instructors to offer expertise and decode relevance without shifting focus from the curriculum to themselves, try telling your significant other about something that happened at work without making yourself the point of the story.

On the way home from PALS, I considered how lucky I was to have had so many outstanding lecturers during my primary EMT and paramedic programs. Although none of my teachers had formal training as educators, they shared qualities that should make some career instructors envious:

Commitment. The best teachers I've known have been "all in"—as dedicated to excellence as the finest EMS providers. So many people are affected by our performance, I can't imagine doing either job without caring about outcomes. Educators on automatic pilot miss almost as much as their students.

Creativity. Some EMS lectures can be pretty boring. Trust me, I've given enough of them. Good instructors try extra hard to punch-up material with imagination and even trickery. I had a teacher who used to write with his left hand once in a while instead of his right, just to see if anyone noticed. Sometimes he'd come to class in homemade costumes to help illustrate the day's lesson. We thought Mr. Clark was crazy, but we sure paid attention to see what stunt he would try next.

Availability. Teaching is one of those occupations, like medicine and law, that doesn't always conform to eight-hour days. When students or patients or clients need you, they usually need you now—not when you're next in your office. Unlike doctors and attorneys, though, most teachers don't have the option of billing for their discretionary time. Excellent educators have to be okay with accommodating pupils' sometimes-frantic, often-inconvenient phone calls, emails, and texts.

Enthusiasm. It's difficult to get excited about presenting dry material after a busy day or night doing your other job, but successful instructors find ways to self-start. Whenever I'd catch myself mumbling to the class about the mysteries of that week's body system, I'd raise my voice a notch, start walking up and down the aisles, and make eye contact with as many students as possible.

Charm. I think it would be hard to thrive as a teacher without a baseline fondness for people. Successful instructors can be serious and even strict while publicly rooting for their students to succeed. Gaining a class's attention without instilling fear often means adding a measure of warmth to each day's lesson plan.

Knowledge. Rule number one of teaching is know the material—trite, perhaps, but I'm betting most of you have endured at least as many unprepared instructors as I have. Spend a little time before class anticipating students' questions.

Experience. You've probably heard the saying "Those who can, do; those who can't, teach." I've seen examples of that, but a more accurate statement, in my opinion, would be "Many who do, can't teach." I think field experience is a necessary but insufficient prerequisite for EMS instructors. Classroom experience—as educator and pupil—is just as important.

Humility. Formal instruction is an exercise requiring mutual respect between teachers and students. That sometimes breaks down when educators wait to show respect until they get it. I've seen much better results when teachers begin their very first lesson with vocabulary, tone, and body language that says "This isn't about me; it's about you mastering the material. I'm going to help you do that."

With self-assured wisdom, we lecture that EMS isn't for everyone. I can almost hear a student's cynical comeback: "Neither is teaching."

Author's Note

Thanks, Bob, Ed, Eric, Paul, and Reeve. I was paying attention even when I looked like I wasn't.

First, I need someone close to tell me that. Next, I'd better suppress a defiant streak I've been known to show, and consider the possibility I've lost my perspective. Then it's time to "reboot" my connection to EMS—to remember I left a perfectly proper but unfulfilling corporate career for the privilege of aiding others. To ignore signs of paroxysmal ambivalence would be disrespectful to those who served in this field before me.

★★★

On July 22, 2007, at Dickey-Stephens Park in Little Rock, Arkansas, Mike Coolbaugh was struck behind the left ear by a baseball hit so hard that even 90 feet away, he had less than half a second to react. That wasn't long enough. The line drive crushed his left vertebral artery, depriving his brain stem of oxygenated blood. Although on-site paramedics, doctors, and nurses—many of whom were paying customers—initiated the most futile of prehospital algorithms within a minute of Coolbaugh's collapse, the consensus is he was dead before he hit the ground.

The Coolbaugh tragedy, while shocking, isn't bigger than baseball. The game goes on with men like Mike who set good examples. His story reminds us that in sports, EMS, or any occupation, dignity isn't measured in dollars, conscientiousness isn't dictated by contracts, and respect for one's profession—despite stress, frustration, malaise, or misfortune—fosters excellence.

Batter up.

A NIGHT AT THE OPRY

2009

A few years ago, my wife and I relocated from New York to Nashville. I had retired—or thought so—after 14 years in EMS and an even longer hitch as a civilian. Lower cost of living, a milder climate, and a leisurely lifestyle were good reasons to head south. I meant to sit on my front porch and watch other people go to work.

It didn't happen that way. I underestimated my attachment to EMS. Nine months of not responding to emergencies was all I could take. My wonky back wouldn't let me return to the streets, so I settled for a part-time position at Opryland, an upscale entertainment complex that's a middle-American Mecca for convention-goers and pleasure-seekers. Less than a year after leaving the northeast, I was a Music City medic.

Tonight, I'm backstage at The Grand Ole Opry, writing this from a small but well-stocked clinic. Yes, I've already done my check-outs, not that it matters much. I rarely see patients who need more than an NSAID. I have a feeling tonight will be different, though. If you'll stay with me, I promise to describe every detail of hearts restarted, lungs re-inflated, and limbs reattached. Hey, you have your protocols, I have mine.

Someone's calling me from the hallway. Maybe I should grab my bag. Maybe I should find my radio. Maybe I should open the door.

Looks like another case of TB—toe blister. I don't mean to boast, but I've seen hundreds of cases down here. TB strikes young women who favor five-inch heels. There is no cure short of sensible shoes.

My patient is a world-class performer with many hit songs. Her voice brings tears to the eyes. So does her blister, apparently. It's beyond my scope of practice to lecture her about foot care. A Band-Aid is the most I can offer without consulting medical control.

As I enjoy the after-action glow of another successful podiatric call, I ponder the possibility of a cardiac arrest in the crowd. I don't know why I torment myself with such medic-unfriendly scenarios. After considering the corn-row seating and narrow aisles at the Opry, I resolve to treat comatose customers as if I've found them in a familiar setting: between a tub and a toilet. With an audience of 3,000. Now I feel better.

There's a knock at the door (I really should prop it open). This is probably the big one. I'm thinking anterolateral-septal-elliptical-geophysical MI with such extreme right axis deviation that it becomes left axis deviation. Or something like that. Someone fetch the spare LIFEPAK battery! And electrodes, lots of electrodes! Boil some water, too! Stat!

Let me preface what happened next with a little background: An old partner of mine once chided me for being so ALS-fixated that I would "hook-up a hangnail." I never had the opportunity to prove her wrong. Until now. Yes, the chief complaint was a hangnail. I swear I didn't overtreat it. It was BLS before ALS all the way. But if that hangnail had become ischemic . . . never mind.

It's getting late. In a region where biscuits and gravy is considered a food group, how does everybody stay so healthy? Doesn't anyone out there need an IV?

Ah, another patient. Sort of. One of the singers managed by my visitor is about to go on stage and needs medication for "frozen vocal cords." Huh? Do they have a protocol for that down here? I knew I shouldn't have skipped the Laryngeal Hypothermia class in medic school. Just as I'm about to admit ignorance, I hear the allegedly mute performer shout, "Forget it, I found some ibuprofen."

Memo to all manufacturers of that wonder drug: Your product could be to frozen vocal cords what aspirin is to MIs.

The show's over, but I see an elderly woman heading straight for my office. Years of experience tell me she's distressed. Cardiac? Could be. Respiratory? Possibly. I can feel the adrenalin (it's right here in my bag, next to the atropine). I crank open the O_2 as my guest crosses the threshold. "Can I help you?" I ask, trying to sound like Marcus Welby mimicking Tennessee Ernie Ford.

"You sure can, doc, if you know where the ladies' room is."

I offer to show her the way and mention I'm not a doctor. At this point, I'm not even sure I'm a medic. I shut the tank and the door behind us.

Okay, maybe entertainment EMS isn't so . . . entertaining. At least I finished my night at the Opry without being crippled, shot at, or slimed. The music was first-rate, and I had time to write this column. There are worse ways to earn a living.

Author's Note

I worked this shift just a few weeks after being hired by Opryland, Nashville's world-class re-sort. I was there for almost six years as a part-time paramedic, alternating between the Grand Ole Opry, The General Jackson riverboat, and Opryland's 2880-room hotel. It never got old standing backstage at the Opry, wondering how a hockey-playing, rock-'n'-rolling engineer/ medic from Boston had become a caregiver to country music's biggest stars.

WITHOUT
SUBSTANCE

2013

I'm happy to say I don't get many calls at home from Alan, my boss—not that I have anything against him. He's a good guy, and we share a lot of interests outside EMS. It's just that I've adopted a no-news-is-good-news outlook that's just as relevant to my work as it is to my colonoscopies.

If I do hear from Alan right before my shift, I almost always know why he's calling: I'm the lucky winner of an all-expenses-paid trip to a Music City lavatory in a Music City laboratory for a drug test. Yee ha.

I support random drug testing in EMS. I see nothing wrong with requiring us to mentate at least as well as the people we treat. Our system of healthcare is scary enough without asking our patients to accommodate dopey medics.

For most of us in EMS, drug tests are as inevitable as recertification. We're not the only ones; some municipalities require all civil servants to be substance-free—at least at the time of hire—and hold members of essential services to even stricter standards. I'm okay with my lifestyle choices being limited by well-intentioned concern for the greater good. The ACLU can sit this one out.

Perhaps the best-known targets of random drug testing are professional athletes, whose specimen regimens are meant to ensure that competitive advantages are congenital, not chemical. I suppose that's important on some level, but I've never felt the outrage of fellow sports fans when some outfielder or midfielder, forward or defender, halfback or fullback gets nabbed by the substance police. I'm more concerned about diminished performance behind steering wheels than enhanced performance on playing fields.

I do believe some professions should be scrutinized more closely. Let's start at the top. Yes, I mean the *very* top: The President of the United States. You think he should have a free pass? Not as long as he has the ability to give dinosaurs a second chance. A hungover paramedic can do some damage, but imagine a return-to-the-planet-of-the-apes scenario triggered by a president on PCPs who pushes the wrong button. I'm not sure, but I think a two-thirds majority in the Senate is needed to tase the chief executive. Don't bet on bipartisan support for that; pre-emptive pee testing would be a lot easier.

Another occupation that cries out for mental-status monitoring is veterinary medicine. I was having a conversation with my cat about this just the other day. Timmy said it was bad enough getting "fixed" when nothing was broken; he shouldn't have had to worry about unsteady hands radicalizing the procedure.

Most people I know seem to deal with drug testing as minor inconveniences—until they get busted. Two ways of ruining your reputation are (1) shopping for shoes while wearing an ankle monitor and (2) failing a drug test.

As a cog in my company's well-care machinery, I've heard my share of excuses from people who test positive for recreational chemicals:

- "I ate poppy seeds."
- "I drank coffee."
- "I drank poppy-flavored coffee".

Please. Save us both the trouble and simply resign in disgrace. Unless you can produce a prescription showing you're under the care of a physician who attended Woodstock, I'm not even listening. Well, maybe a little. I admit I'm concerned about mistakes being made whenever *I'm* tested. I watch *Law & Order*. I've seen how one unscrupulous lab technician can ruin the lives of hundreds of innocent citizens right before burdening our justice system with appeals of every guilty verdict since Cain v. Abel. *Res ipsa loquitur*, K.

What if I'm unlucky enough to draw a righteously indignant lab tech with sloppy work habits and sociopathic tendencies? It could happen. Would I still be able to argue my urine is clean—relative to other urine, I mean? Do I offer another sample? Submit to a lie detector? I've heard you can't trust those machines. How am I supposed to convince someone I'm not lying about not lying?

These are issues that occupy my mind far more often than eight out of ten dentists recommend. I think I need a prescription for something that looks like aspirin, works like Valium, tastes like Ex-Lax, but is chemically similar to, say, oregano.

It would be very important not to mix those up.

THE LITTLE PICTURE

2015

Pay attention!

I must have said that to my daughter dozens of times during her primary-school years, when her mind wandered instead of staying close to the rest of her. Nothing unusual about that; I've seen pulse checks last longer than kids' attention spans. When children do focus, it's usually on their terms, and only until something better comes along.

I wasn't worried Becky might one day "overdose" on concentration—that she'd be so intent on completing a single task, she'd lose track of everything else going on around her. Only one person I know has that problem:

My name is Mike, and I have tunnel vision.

There, I've said it. Those of you who used to ride with me may already know. If not, ask my wife. She'll tell you about the time she was waving at me while we were treating an elderly male in a filthy apartment. At least I thought she was waving. Turns out she was swatting—gnats, enough of them to have carried the patient to the ambulance themselves, she told me later. I was too busy taking vitals and wondering why no one was helping me. I swear I didn't notice any life forms smaller than Helen.

Then there's the morning I asked her if she'd be making coffee—while I was holding a cup of it. No doubt I was thinking great thoughts at the time, but that didn't discourage Helen from wondering aloud if I'd suffered any concussions she wasn't aware of.

Tunnel vision is a tendency to miss something really important while fixating on something less important. The narrower the "tunnel," the more you miss. If there were a Borg scale for tunnel vision, with "1" as a tunnel the size of your basic school corridor and "10" as the inside of an 8.5 endotracheal tube, I'd register about a "7"—the cramped sewer pipe that guy crawled through in *The Shawshank Redemption*. I can get *very* preoccupied. If you find me unresponsive, please don't pronounce me until you're sure I'm not just concentrating.

I pay too much attention to lots of things—like how I'm writing. I mean right now. My obsession with wordplay is an excellent example of one man's focus on the *little* picture. Does *little* sound better than *small*? Was *cramped* a good adjective for a sewer pipe? Don't worry, my editor and I will have it straightened out by the time you read this.

Sometimes tunnel vision really means *tunnel* vision, as in the underground kind. I'm remembering one of those otherworldly "man under" calls in the New York City subway system. I was so fascinated at being track-level, I forgot to ask whether the juice had been shut off until I was straddling the third rail. I didn't dare resume a position of comfort until a train worker stepped on the rail to prove it was safe. What a guy. I bet if he were a medic, he'd cardiovert himself just to show a patient it doesn't hurt much.

It isn't hard to spot medics with tunnel vision. They're the ones on scene mumbling "just one more try" while pointing unsheathed angiocaths at patients' exposed limbs. It's probably best not to get in their way until their IV attempts have taken longer than a trip to the hospital would have, or no one can remember why an IV was even needed.

I'm pretty sure medics with tunnel vision get lots of what-is-your-problem looks from partners. I wouldn't know because tunnel vision prevents me from noticing. To those of you who enjoy rolling your eyes at someone else's plight, let me just say . . . uh . . . I can't remember what I was going to say. I'm still thinking about that tunnel-vision Borg scale, and whether a "10" should be a 14-gauge catheter instead of an ET tube. Just give me a minute . . .

Tunnel vision isn't all bad. Sufferers tend to conduct *very* thorough patient interviews—about childhood illnesses, recurring dreams, favorite colors—and can complete important tasks without being distracted by loud music or funnel clouds. It's that short-term disconnect that occasionally compromises big-picture priorities, like survival.

The only hope for families with the tunnel-vision gene, I suppose, is for parents of afflicted children to employ a rather unconventional form of negative reinforcement:

"Pay *less* attention!"

Author's Note

I think I've gotten better at tunnel vision . . . I mean having less of it—better at having less tunnel vision, as opposed to being better at having more of it, which would be bad and not quite like English.

Never mind.

HELPING HANDS

2009

I'd like to introduce you to a friend of mine. His name is Sal. Some of your patients may already know him, or someone like him. I hope so.

Sal isn't a firefighter, a paramedic, or an EMT. Nor is he a PA, RN, or MD. He isn't a big fan of PDAs, KEDs, SUVs, or AC/DC. I think he's OK with MLB and the AARP.

Sal is a Marine because there's no such thing as an ex-Marine. He's been answering alarms for a suburban New York EMS agency for 40 years. Do you know what I was doing 40 years ago? Neither do I. Something involving English or History or Algebra, I suppose.

When Sal started in EMS, ambulance-based ALS was as controversial as billion-dollar bank bailouts. Sal spent some time as a "para-paramedic" before prehospital levels of practice were well-defined. He enjoyed providing patient care and didn't mind driving those Cadillac hearses. Sal liked EMS so much, he did it every day. For free. Yes, Sal's a volunteer.

I met Sal in the early 90s when I had no training but lots of interest in EMS. He helped convince me there are worse ways to spend one's time than aiding the sick and injured. Sal had to remind me of that many years later when survival-to-discharge became an elusive goal and I contemplated a return to corporate life.

Like many of you, I participate in Web-based EMS forums. I've read several threads debating the merits of paid-versus-volunteer personnel. I've rarely seen such a contentious topic, but the online opinions sound familiar. As an EMS administrator during the first half of this decade, I worked with dozens of volunteer agencies supplemented by paid staffers. The issues haven't changed:

Training

I sense a concern that volunteers aren't trained to the same standards as paid personnel, yet I'm unaware of any states where *volunteer* is a prefix or suffix appended to EMS certifications. EMTs are EMTs whether or not they receive W-2 forms.

Paid services don't have a monopoly on continuing education, either. The only time I was required to undergo monthly training was as a volunteer. None of my employers have insisted on anything more than state-mandated biennial or triennial refreshers. Also, when I decided to upgrade from EMT to paramedic, my volunteer agency paid the bill. That would not have happened at any of my salaried postings.

Competence

What makes people competent in any field? Education? Experience? Character? Talent? I don't think any of those attributes are restricted to paid personnel. When I was responsible for evaluating thousands of prehospital cases a year, I found no correlation between quality of care and compensation. The most accurate predictor of performance was experience.

Do you remember how frustrating it was to apply for your first mortgage, credit card, or car loan, only to be told you needed credit to get credit? EMS novices are victims of a similar catch-22 when they're informed they won't be hired without experience. Volunteering is a good way to bridge that gap.

The ways managers of both paid and volunteer EMS agencies assist, measure, and critique subordinates' management of prehospital challenges contribute even more to competence, I believe, than the number of years practitioners have served in the field.

Encroachment

Volunteers are seen by some as limiting opportunities for paid providers. The logic is that municipalities have no incentive to add EMS jobs or increase wages if well-meaning citizens are willing to answer alarms for free.

I agree the public plays a role in determining our employment opportunities, but it's not just about money. The issue should be who can deliver the highest quality of care and best service for the lowest fee. Some jurisdictions feel volunteers offer the most favorable price/performance ratio. I discovered as much when I tried to convince an isolated, well-to-do community at the edge of an all-volunteer district that a dedicated paid service would offer more experienced personnel and faster response. Cost wasn't a concern for this upper-class enclave, yet the village rejected my proposal because they were satisfied with the level of care they were getting from unpaid personnel. Perceived value mattered more than provider pedigree.

Attitude

I used to generalize that volunteers possessed a sense of entitlement their paid colleagues did not. I must admit, I've met many members of both groups who crave respect and privilege to compensate for on-the-job risks and disruption in family life. I'm not sure how much of that longing is evident to the public, but I know this: I'd rather be treated by a considerate, conscientious volunteer than a churlish career medic.

One of the great healers of the last 2,009 years asserted that charity should be offered anonymously. Thousands of volunteers do this every day. Should their abilities be scrutinized? No more or less than the rest of us. However, the existence of EMS as a vocation doesn't diminish the intrinsic goodness of volunteering, nor does it preclude acknowledgment of contributors like Sal.

Author's Note

Sal died three years after I wrote this. I've known a few men like Sal, but none better.

THE MOST INTERESTING MEDIC IN THE WORLD

2012

My favorite TV commercials are the beer ads starring actor
Jonathan Goldsmith as "the most interesting man in the world."
It's not the product I'm attracted to; it's the character. Who wouldn't
want to be interesting to everyone?

Twenty years as a sportswriter/engineer/manager/consultant
didn't do that for me. I could tell by the gratuitous curiosity and
thousand-yard stares from cocktail-party minglers whenever we'd
discuss work. I don't blame them; I wasn't all that interested in what
I did for a living, either.

Later, I discovered paramedics aren't rated any higher on the
I-want-to-be-like-him scale than my prior occupations were. Most
of us in EMS aren't interesting enough to impress anyone we're not
treating. It's not our personalities, it's our work. We'd be rock stars if
we handled as many shootings per shift as our stunt doubles depict
on TV. Instead, we spend most of our field time treating formidable
but fundamentally dull diseases like diabetes and COPD. The better
people understand our routine, the less interesting we seem.

Sometimes, we hurt our cause by substituting simplistic expressions for more thorough explanations of what we do. "Jump-starting
the heart" is an example. If I told my neighbor I do that, he'd probably think, *What's the big deal? I jump-started my wife's car the other
day.* I bet he'd be more impressed if I said I depolarized my patient's

myocardium so intrinsic pacemakers could resume normal activity. He might also keep his children away from me.

If the most interesting man in the world were a paramedic—in his spare time, so it didn't get in the way of skydiving or bull-fighting—I suspect he'd maintain enough of a mystique to charm the public. I can imagine him being interviewed after yet another save:

"I don't always defibrillate," he'd offer, coyly, "but when I do, I prefer rectilinear biphasic waveforms." I know *I'd* be thinking there's no cooler EMS provider on the planet. Soon the legend would transcend the man and we'd be hearing these stories about The Most Interesting Medic in the World:

- He delivers babies with Apgar scores of 11.
- Patients offer to name their illnesses after him.
- His chest compressions are so effective, 60 a minute are enough.
- He has more standing orders than his medical director.
- Hospitals divert patients to him.
- He secretes his own disinfectant.
- Nursing homes prepare elaborate patient histories just for him.
- He finishes late calls early.
- He's the only medic certified in IPTLS (Inter-Planetary Trauma Life Support).
- His IVs are never removed by hospital staff.
- He verifies endotracheal tubes inserted by anesthesiologists.
- He diagnoses STEMIs from artifact.
- Ambulances circle his scene until summoned by him.
- He eats and sleeps just to be polite.
- He's the only paramedic to hold EMT-MD certification.
- His arrival makes scenes safe.

(Yes, I realize the most interesting medic in the world might be female, but I had to pick a pronoun. Have mercy.)

It's fun to fantasize, but reality intervenes whenever we respond to the ultra-high-definition world of live trauma and disease. Suddenly, the stakes change: We don't have to be interesting, just good. When people talk about us, we'd be happy if they just said:

- He'd make a good teacher.
- He comforts kids when they cry.

- He's a patient advocate even when the system makes that hard.
- I felt so much better after talking to him.
- He's gentle with the truth when the news is bad.
- He eases pain, even when that's all he can do.
- That's one service I don't mind paying taxes for.
- I hope he's here the next time I need help.

EMS providers may not be interesting, but we're necessary and often effective. As much as anyone, we make direct contributions to the neediest segments of society. We wish we were as admired as athletes and actors—who doesn't?—but we understand that our jobs are to work behind the scenes. We willingly trade fame for inconspicuous competence. We'd settle for a few fans who want to be like us, even if they don't want to be us.

Stay trusty, my friends.

Author's Note

This TV commercial stayed on the air until they tried replacing Goldsmith with a less-interesting actor. It was like swapping Randolph Mantooth for Pee Wee Herman.

ON FALLIBILITY

2015

Not long ago, a dear friend who'd been a patient of mine was diagnosed with an aggressive cancer. As soon as I heard, I thought
of the last time I'd treated her and wondered if there were any connection between her illness that day and the hideous disease that had
almost certainly entered her bones by then. So much of her complaint had seemed predictable at the time, based on her pre-cancer
history, that I'd neglected to ask myself a very important question:
What else could it be?

Zebras—we're talking zebras, not horses; the same zebras we're
not supposed to think of when we hear something that sounds like
them. It's a good rule, the one about hoofbeats meaning horses, until
it's not. So many rules in EMS are like that. We might as well replace
them all with *Do the right thing*, or *Try to do the right thing*, or maybe
just *Try*.

Trying is easier than doing when you have limitations. I have
many, according to The Lovely Helen. I don't disagree, but prefer to
console myself with the expectation of getting smarter as I get older.
I'm not sure how many years that will take. So far, I can tell you it's
not mistakes that decrease with age; it's second chances.

For many years, I made the most of my mulligans and resolved
any lingering cognitive dissonance about choosing an EMS career
versus a longer corporate one by vowing to do better on my next call.
Now, there are no more next calls, no more opportunities to improve.

The nastiest part is wondering how much difference a smarter
medic would have made. I can't think of an analogy in the 9-5 world.
I mean, how much sympathy would you have for a boardroom full of
executives second-guessing their sales forecasts?

There were missed opportunities during the 9-1-1 years. I'm
thinking of a patient for whom breathing had become an unnatural
act. How long before I got there, I can't say. Was her brain still capable

of intricate function? I don't know that, either. Intubation might have helped if I'd found the right hole.

I've considered the notion that it was "her time"—what we now call *qualitative futility*. Who knows, she may have frolicked into the light fully aware of my fallibility. I'll never know.

Part of the problem, I think, is the way we measure ourselves, which is not much at all. The only routine clinical feedback I had during most of my career is when my patients got at least some of their circulation back. We called that a save and there was much gladness, even if saved patients died a few moments later. With pulses as our *raison d'être*, no wonder epi was such a popular drug.

I'd like to think EMS is about results and pulses are only part of the picture, but then how do we explain this missive from the American Heart Association to ACLS students:

"Your success will not be measured by whether a cardiac arrest patient lives or dies, but rather by the fact that you tried and worked well together as a team. Simply by taking action, making an effort, and trying to help, you will be judged a success."

Maybe that's why doctors seemed so understanding when they pronounced my patients.

Is there a trend here? Does trying hard override failure? If so, I'm golden.

Or perhaps anxiety about missed opportunities to excel is just part of what author, actor and director Miranda July calls feeling "secretly fraudulent." Have you ever felt that way—as if one of these days, people will discover you don't belong in EMS?

If so, retirement brings relief. At first.

Author's Note

That statement by the AHA still bothers me. I'm not a fan of the everybody-gets-a-trophy mindset, nor do I think most "saves" are worth special attention.

SELECTIVE
SERVICE

2015

Sometime during the first half-century of EMS, the public we serve got the notion we're doing them a favor. Consider the following example:

Early in the post-Y2K decade, I was channel surfing at home between shifts at my favorite hospital-based EMS agency when I spotted a county official on a call-in TV talk show—a format long since replaced by exposés about naked-and-afraid housewives who hoard. I recognized him as someone whose chain of command I was part of, so I stopped clicking long enough to hear him take a call from a resident who complained about a slow response by fire or EMS to some sort of emergency.

There had been lots of debate at my job about response times: how they should be measured, who should measure them, what reasonable goals were, etc. Now I was curious about how my boss's boss's boss was going to respond to the televised complaint. Addressing the caller, he replied, "When *you* start getting up in the middle of the night to answer emergencies, then you can criticize."

Wow—that was like saying you have to be a chef to send back an undercooked steak. Surely there would be an outcry from indignant viewers who shouldn't have to be paramedics in order to call for one.

There was no outcry. Not even a murmur. It was as if the government guy had spoken the truth, or at least what viewers thought was the truth.

That talk show reminded me of two things: Never underestimate the entertainment value of live TV, and essential services are considered by many to be favors granted by those who are paid to deliver them. It embarrasses me to acknowledge that some who share the latter view are EMS providers.

On my worst days, I've behaved as if my patients were privileged to have me. I didn't mean to; it just happened sometimes when I wasn't properly motivated to be a rescuer, like the time the husband of a pleasantly confused patient tried to tell me which hospital his wife preferred. I cut him off and told him we're going to the closest ED, even though the patient's stable condition gave us more flexibility than that. The husband smiled and shrugged, sidestepping an opportunity to point out that I was exhibiting an aberrant form of role reversal: a public servant who wanted to be served. We both knew our destination was convenient for me, not for my patient.

Speaking of convenience, I don't know how I got the notion I was owed any. So many of us go into EMS to avoid environmentally controlled jobs with mind-numbing routines. It shouldn't have been hard for me to roll the dice and let my patient pick the hospital.

There is no shortage of excuses for the entitlement we feel when we "qualify" patients for assistance we're required to offer. Being overworked and underpaid certainly makes it easier for us to justify, at least to ourselves, the need for a defensive posture. An us-against-the-world attitude leaves little room for courtesy, though, and turns us into caricatures of the public servants we're supposed to be.

That explains how EMS providers get confused about who's serving whom, but why does the public cut us so much slack for acting that way?

One reason is that people don't know much about what we do. Another is that people don't *want* to know much about what we do.

I think most of the public is comfortable regarding EMS as a black box with mysterious mechanisms that somehow cause ambulances to appear at medical emergencies. That knowledge gap is an issue for another day. Meanwhile, if you've not only carried a stretcher but occupied one, you know how disruptive emergent illness or injury can be for the sufferer, and how welcome the slightest courtesies can be to patients transitioning from self-sufficient to dependent.

Suppose those of us in EMS really are special, with nobility fused to our DNA like wings on angels. What better way to show we've earned our blue blood than by *delivering* service, instead of expecting it?

Even if it means getting up in the middle of the night.

Author's Note

Don't get me started on service providers who don't provide service.

Too late.

At 68, I feel I get profiled as a semi-lucid senior who inconveniences the service sector with my mere presence. It's annoying when that happens in a supermarket, and dangerous when it happens on an ambulance.

CRITICAL THINKING

2013

I'm trying to remember when I started caring about making mistakes. I think it was the first time I read a story aloud in Mrs. Hancock's first grade class. I don't remember the title; possibly *Dick and Jane Build an Air-Raid Shelter*, given late 50s sensibilities. I just know I wanted to do well—not to impress my teacher, but because reading the right way made me feel better about myself.

Messing up sentences embarrassed me more than being corrected. When I did mispronounce words, I sensed Mrs. Hancock's feedback was well-intended, and discovered if I paid attention to her, I'd make fewer errors and go home happier. Even as a six-year-old, I was starting to understand the value of constructive criticism.

The consequences of screwing up are much greater for me now than in 1959, but I still feel the same about mistakes: If I can't avoid them, I want to at least learn from them so I don't make the same ones again. I was happy to see that point emphasized by someone called Rocketmedic40 on a popular EMS website. (Memo to readers: I don't know Rocketmedic40's gender, so I'm going to use the one I'm most familiar with.)

Rocketmedic40, a paramedic student from Yukon, Oklahoma, was writing about his first "code save." He began by admitting deficiencies: uncertain airway management, tunnel vision compromising resource allocation, and delayed medication administration. Next, he summarized strengths: IO access, effective CPR, and timely defibrillation. He closed by giving credit to colleagues for the favorable outcome. Overall, it was a pretty impressive analysis from someone new to running calls. Such a level-headed self-critique is rare.

Perhaps Rocketmedic40's preceptor would have added equally constructive comments, but in my experience, tentative, ambiguous feedback from supervisors is more likely. The problem, I think, is a bias not to offend, rather than to educate—a fallacy that discourages quality improvement. Let me offer an example:

In the late '90s, a law was passed in the state where I worked that mandated quarterly reviews of prehospital care. The guidelines were broad, leaving it up to administrators to decide the nature and scope of calls examined. Confidentiality was considered one of the biggest obstacles—more for providers than patients. There were concerns that criticism might discourage or even offend caregivers, many of whom were serving as volunteers. Reviewers, blinded to the identities of crews, often generated recommendations to the entire community of prehospital practitioners based on the actions of only a few, while missing opportunities to offer meaningful, individualized positive and negative reinforcement.

How do you feel when everyone in your department gets a memo criticizing the group for an error made by an individual? When that happens to me, I might think the published offense sounds like something I did; more likely, I'll wonder why I'm being remediated for something I didn't do. In either case, the value of the message is diminished by dilution of reinforcement to avoid conflict—one of the most common management blunders I've witnessed in 45 years of employment.

What can EMS providers do to compensate for vague or misdirected feedback? I think we should favor the sort of self-critique Rocketmedic40 demonstrated—not to replace external appraisals, but to complement them. Beware of these obstacles, though:

Ego. Conceding mistakes requires a suspension of disbelief our egos don't always permit. Robert Townsend, author of 1970's seminal *Up the Organization*, suggests we set good examples not just by admitting our own errors, but by publicizing them. That encourages others to see the constructive side of fallibility.

Difficulty applying new knowledge. It's hard to judge your own performance in an unfamiliar environment. If you're new to EMS, you won't have adequate experience for a comprehensive self-assessment. Consider less technical parts of the job—e.g., if you were your patient, how would you feel about the care you just received?

Misunderstanding the process. It's not enough to recognize our mistakes; quality assurance dictates we modify our flawed behavior and see if results improve. That back end of the QA/QI loop is often omitted.

The ability to gauge one's own performance—calmly, unemotionally, and as objectively as possible—is a survival skill learned over time. It takes practice and a willingness to see ourselves as works in progress. The payoff is gaining insight from your harshest critic: you.

EMS.O.S.

2015

For years, I've been trying to justify my appreciation of The Three Stooges—mostly to The Lovely Helen, who claims the Stooges are proof the alleged 5% difference between human and chimpanzee DNA is more like 4% in men. To my wife I say, wake up and go to sleep.

"Getting" the Stooges is a Mars/Venus thing. On behalf of my fellow Martians who happen to be in the patient-processing business, I've figured out how to make Moe, Larry, and Curly almost as relevant to EMS as Johnny and Roy. But first, some background:

I've noticed discussions on EMS web sites about use of code words to request help in the field urgently and secretly. I can relate. I used to annoy my partners at Opryland with hypothetical scenarios about sedate guests suddenly going postal. What if a presenting lunatic insists I treat him for an allergic reaction to, say, gun powder, and then refuses the SWAT team AMA? Am I supposed to look for an opportunity to disarm him with my penlight? "Sir, I just need to check your pupils for a few minutes—slowly, very slowly, while you're getting sleepy, so sleepy . . ." I don't think so.

A better solution would be a stealthy signal known only by my agency, its members, their spouses, and Facebook friends, meaning *help me right now or I will haunt you the rest of your life.* Just put it in the back of the employee handbook under a heading that only EMS people would look at—something like *Photo of Human Eyeball Clawed by Rabid Chipmunk.*

Look no further than The Three Stooges for a precedent. They had to deal with imminent badness in their 1950 short, *Studio Stoops.*

Moe and Larry are in a room, hiding from gangsters. As Larry leaves, he tells Moe, "When I come back, I'll give you the password."

"Brilliant. What'll it be?" asks Moe.

"Open the door."

That still cracks me up, but the idea of prearranged words or phrases in EMS to limit danger is worth considering. I don't remember being in a situation where I needed that, but I came close, twice, when patients who told me they were ex-cons objected rather vigorously to being examined in a small room with a closed door. Okay, so maybe I shouldn't have referred to my LIFEPAK 10 as "Old Sparky," but hey, live and learn.

If we're going to do this, we need to decide on the type of signal we'll use. Consider these possibilities:

10-Codes

Almost every department has them or used to have them. The best thing about 10-codes is they'll sound plausible to psychopaths.

The problem is consistency; there is none. I've worked in systems where 10-1, 10-3, 10-13 and 10-24 each meant *help in the name of all that is holy*, but 10-13 might be the code for ordering a pepperoni pizza in some places.

Secret Words

I'm thinking they should be part of routine transmissions—something like "Medic Rubin to Base, show me back in service *PUH-LEECE*." Or "Hospital X, I'm inbound with a *morderiske galning*." That's Danish for *homicidal maniac*. Studies show very few sociopaths speak Danish.

Telltale Phrases

One approach would be to involve a significant other, as in, "Hey, honey, just called to say how much I enjoyed watching *Real Housewives* with you." Helen would know right away I was in trouble, or suffering from a berry aneurysm. Either way, she'd call 9-1-1.

An alternative would be to keep it strictly business: "Base, just wondering when that shipment of bretylium will be in." Heh heh, got you there, Mr. Bad Guy . . . unless you happen to be one of my deranged ex-partners.

Absurd Protocols

You could disguise your crisis code as a medical control option. Medical control would figure out something's wrong if you asked for, say, a chamomile infusion or a porridge challenge. I bet they'd send help after they yanked your card.

Nonverbal Signals

How about keying *S.O.S.* through our radios? Oh, so Morse code isn't part of *your* curriculum? Fine, then just keep pressing PTT to the beat of "Stayin' Alive."

Cell phones might work if we could operate them like spies do in the movies—by feel, from a pocket. The idea would be to discreetly send a canned text message; something like "I'm being kidnapped by a patient who's fondling my stethoscope." Not sure about that one; Helen might think it's just another pathetic excuse for being late.

Nyuk, nyuk, nyuk.

Author's Note

I'm not sure if this is good news or bad, but I enjoy watching The Three Stooges even more as I get older. Helen says it's because I'm temperamental—95% temper and 5% mental ("Saved by the Bell", 1939).

A CRY FOR HELP

2013

What impression would you have of a patient with this chief complaint?

"Something happened yesterday that just put me over the edge. I need to sleep, see my friends, see my fiancée.

"I want to make others happy and put their happiness before my own. I always have. But I guess I need to find a balance.

"Maybe it was just a bad day, but after today I feel like I've had enough."

You'd be concerned, wouldn't you? Even if the subject's affect were unremarkable, you'd probably label your patient potentially unstable and conclude there isn't anything in your drug box to address those signs and symptoms.

Here's another unsettling presentation:

"Life to me is a game of many turns, hills, tests and sacrifices I must face. I've been to war and I've made it back home, but making it back home is what I would give up to have the friends I've lost be able to come back home to their families.

"I've been told money means more to me than love. That's one reason I look at life differently today. When the day comes that I must leave the life I'm living, the only question I have for myself is, did I live life the way I wanted to, or did I live the life someone else wanted me to?"

Note the signs of sadness, loss, lack of focus, and perhaps even suicidal ideation in this patient's self-assessment. I don't know about you, but I'd be wondering how dangerous he might be to himself and others.

These quotations, which I've edited for brevity and confidentiality, aren't from patients; they're from EMS providers—people like you and me experiencing, at the very least, what the first EMT characterized as a "bad day," or perhaps something much worse. I mention our fraternal connection with those sufferers only to dispel the notion that we are somehow above public displays of misery.

I see signs of profound despair on EMS forums several times a year, and even more frequently on generic media like Facebook. They make me wonder if those same social networks I've often criticized might have value as surrogate confidants. I'd like to believe no form of digitized communication is as effective as face-to-face conversation, but perhaps I'm being old-fashioned. I see dozens of postings each week that seem to be cathartic for the originators based on the reinforcing tone of ensuing dialogues.

Sometimes, though, there is a sense of desperation that supplants the recreational tenor of posts. I'm not talking about rhetorical references to global warming or indignant exposés of allegedly unfair bosses; I mean gut-wrenching expressions of emotional distress that challenge even the most impervious EMS veteran to sit idly by. Such anguish from colleagues may be particularly unsettling, but a victim's occupation shouldn't determine whether we pay attention.

We're trained to recognize many types of illness. How should we react to the kind that's hard to measure clinically and occurs at such great distances, we have no duty to engage?

Note signs of distress. Pay particular attention to provocative message headers and topics, like "I'm Done" or "It's Over." Cries for help aren't always frantic; often, they sound more like dispassionate determination to act.

Get involved. You don't need permission or protocols for this step. Initiate contact privately—even if the post was public—and indicate a willingness to talk. Show concern, but don't be quick to claim you understand the sufferer's mindset. Patient listening is often more helpful than generic advice.

Let someone know. Most of us don't have the training to handle psychiatric emergencies alone. Explore local resources with your correspondent and consider highlighting the distress call to a forum moderator.

Follow up. Check back with the subject a few days after your initial dialogue. Be particularly sensitive to expressions of hopelessness (e.g., "Nobody cares"), hypothetical questions about medications or weapons, and rambling, disorganized rants.

I'm not suggesting we dial 9-1-1 every time we encounter a "people suck" post. Sometimes, simply having an outlet for frustration allows our on-line neighbors to maintain balance in their stressful environments. Consider, though, the steps we routinely take in the field to err on the side of caution. None of us wants to confront what could have been done.

Author's Note

Stress in EMS is a much more common topic today than it was in 2013. Although I think PTSD is sometimes diagnosed prematurely, I'd rather assume the worst and offer conflicted colleagues high-frequency listening.

HARD TO BELIEVE

2011

I first heard of "evidence-based medicine" during an ACLS class in the mid '90s. We had started the day honing intubation and CPR, then took our seats for the didactic portion of the program. Our instructor credited EBM with changing the way we manage cardiac arrests; for example, discouraging routine use of sodium bicarbonate—treatment that had been considered a standard of care for two decades. He also lauded bretylium's unique "chemical defibrillation" properties, and suggested we make space in our drug bags for high-dose epinephrine. The message to a roomful of novice ALS providers was clear: Driven by the scientific method, EMS was discarding antiquated procedures in favor of leading-edge innovations.

Fast forward to 2000: EBM was discrediting bretylium, high-dose epi, and almost every other drug once thought to promote cardiac arrest survival. Five years later, CPR supplanted pulse checks as the first post-defibrillation step. In 2010, continuous chest compressions leap-frogged airway management and ventilation on the American Heart Association's BLS algorithm, forcing us to relearn "The ABCs" as "The CABs." Also, "large differences in direction and effect between results from the laboratory and those derived from clinical trials" indicated we should take another look at bicarb.

Why so many contradictions in care? Are old studies flawed? Has EBM matured? After reading Jonah Lehrer's "The Truth Wears Off" in December 13th's *The New Yorker*, I think the problem might be EBM itself.

Lehrer labels "replicability"—confirmation of findings by multiple investigators—as "the foundation of modern research," then uses a 2005 *JAMA* review of 49 groundbreaking clinical trials to show how elusive replicability can be. Of 34 studies repeated, only 20 showed comparable results. Lehrer suggests several reasons:

Selective reporting. Often a consequence of subconscious bias rather than willful deceit, selective reporting is more likely when research involves subjective criteria—e.g., appearance, odor, texture. However, even quantitative studies can be compromised by scientists' prior beliefs. It's human nature to prefer results that prove us right.

Selective publishing. Of the 49 trials *JAMA* cited, 45 supported initial hypotheses. Even if we give researchers the benefit of the doubt by assuming their theories are correct 70% of the time, the chances of being right on at least 45 of 49 consecutive, independent occasions are less than 3 in 10,000. A more likely explanation is that authors, publishers, and readers of research often ignore negative findings.

Statistical anomalies. The ongoing debate about global warming reminds us that correlated data—even lots of it— doesn't necessarily forecast long-term trends. Sometimes our conclusions are based on aberrations—chance occurrences that even out over a very long time.

It's not just evidence-based *medicine* we're questioning; evidence of all kinds is on trial. No wonder my Google search for "not well understood" yielded 23 million hits. How, then, should we react to the premise that it's hard to prove anything?

As an engineer, I'm frightened by that prospect. I spent 4 years in college and 18 in business solving hundreds, maybe thousands of problems based on generally accepted principles of energy and motion, all of which were even more entrenched than, say, prophylactic aspirin for MIs (one of the 49 studies highlighted by *JAMA*). Now, I'm reading about discrepancies in the behavior of planets and stars that contradict the work of Newton and Einstein. I can handle doubts about bicarb, but *gravity*?

Conversely, as a medic, I'm not surprised by Lehrer's piece. Each major modification in prehospital care I've witnessed during 19 years in EMS has been accompanied by caveats from more experienced colleagues. That doesn't mean every revised recommendation was ill-conceived, but now I know I was wrong to assume opponents of our industry's "enhancements" were merely resistant to change. Maybe they found a workable, middle ground between evidence-based and "experience-based" medicine.

In the mid-'90s, my colleague, Kevin, expressed surprise at new restrictions on use of MAST trousers. A veteran of NYC★EMS, Kevin recalled countless victims of penetrating trauma who had regained pulses after MAST application. I remember being skeptical because research had shown that raising BPs in patients with open wounds simply caused them to exsanguinate faster. That's still plausible; so is the notion that Kevin's experience contributed more to the care of select patients than all the MAST experiments ever done.

There's another reason I'm rethinking EBM-driven protocols: Five minutes into a recent cardiac arrest, with v-fib refractory to two shocks and CPR, I inserted an OPA. My elderly patient gagged, converted to a sinus rhythm, woke up, and wanted to know why I thought he needed an ambulance.

Was it timing? Luck? A subtle shift in Nashville's magnetic field? Should we resurrect two 20-year-old studies linking vagal stimulation to a rise in v-fib threshold?

I don't know. I'm still contemplating CPR without gravity.

Author's Note

I can't believe I bought into the 2011 notion that global warming is a "statistical anomaly." Yup, that's what I called it, with all the audacity of a medic pushing high-dose epi.

LETTING THE DAYS GO BY

2015

*And you may find yourself in a beautiful house, with a
beautiful wife
And you may ask yourself—well . . . how did I get here?*

—"Once in a Lifetime," Talking Heads

Forty years ago last month, my wife and I got married—not to
each other, which is why September was more about coincidence
than celebration for us. Still, it's an opportunity to look back once
more and wonder how The Lovely Helen and I ended up in EMS, in
EMS together, and just plain together.

Helen once said she probably wouldn't have dated me if we'd met
outside of EMS. I'd like to think she was hinting at the magnificence
of paramedics, but she was more likely contemplating how boring I
must have been as an engineer—my prior occupation. I think I could
have won her over even then with the right combination of charm
and Quaaludes.

Meeting Helen during my fourth year in EMS was almost as important to me as being in EMS. I say "almost" because in 1995, *nothing* was more important to me than EMS—not family or money or
even living until morning. I'm not proud of those feelings. I needed
someone like Helen to take hold of me, look me in the eyes, and ask,
"Are you mental?"

I could see right away Helen was more of a natural caregiver than
I was. I suppose we both got into EMS for the same reason—to seek
comfort by giving it—but I tended to focus on therapeutics while

Helen could sense a broader range of patients' needs. More than once, I saw signs and symptoms I was about to treat subside after nothing more than a pleasant conversation between Helen and the sufferer. Who *wouldn't* want to know Helen better?

Friendship with Helen came with conditions I thought were pretty unreasonable at the time—like having to keep commitments outside of EMS, even if that meant answering one less call. I remember an evening when we were supposed to meet for dinner, but I agreed to cover a shift for a colleague at the last minute. Helen gave me the impression I was a jerk by saying something like, "You're a jerk." Clearly, I would have to treat Helen at least as well as I did people who dialed 9-1-1.

Conventional wisdom states coworkers should avoid romancing each other. Personal problems often become workplace problems that compromise productivity and perhaps even safety. That's why many organizations have written policy restricting friendship to platonic fondness. I agree with the logic.

But logic turns out to have little to do with anything romantic. Companies that try to limit employees' appreciation of each other confuse the way things are with the way things ought to be. You can't legislate feelings. Helen and I came together despite mostly well-meaning advice that we shouldn't.

EMS turns out to be a pretty good training ground for relationships. Having a great partner is a lot like having a successful marriage. Making the transition from the former to the latter is easier and more realistic, I think, than any other way of getting to know a future spouse.

So what do you do when you and your partner develop a connection that stretches beyond the workplace? You keep taking care of your patients competently and unspectacularly, that's what. Being anything less than excellent at your jobs gives skeptics an excuse to say, "I told you so." And being discreet isn't only good business; it's good manners. Nobody wants to hear how much you like each other.

Then there's the point when you "get involved." The sky looks bluer, the daily commute seems shorter, and whatever still bothers you isn't as bad as it used to be. Those are nice-to-have moments, but the real payoff of a loving relationship is its constancy when everything else seems to be changing. As Helen and I age and deal with cumulative losses—family, friends, fitness—we depend on one sure thing: each other. Some partners never develop that trust. Some couples never develop that trust.

For Helen and me, it's the same as it ever was.

PRACTICING MEDICINE

2009

My boss, Kevin, is not an excitable man. I know this because I've occasionally tormented him for the sole purpose of escalating our North-South rivalry. Other than suggesting I could be replaced by someone much younger, he's been imperturbable. That's why I was intrigued by his animated demeanor one day last month.

"Did you hear about the arrest?" he asked. I told him I hadn't. "Well, I got a tube. First one since I've been here [almost two years]." I didn't ask about the outcome; I knew Kevin would have led with that if there had been a happy ending. We briefly debated whether Mr. Miller or Mr. Macintosh had designed the better tool for airway penetration before concluding that the intubation of Kevin's lifeless, morbidly obese patient was, at the very least, "good practice."

When I use that term to characterize my intervention in someone's misfortune, I worry about sounding like a carnival sideshow barker, treating tragedy as opportunity instead of adversity. I don't actually hope for illness or injury. What I mean is that I rely on the inevitability of trauma and disease to hone my craft; that my therapeutic skills will erode without repetition and reinforcement from favorable outcomes. In short, I need the practice.

A benign, productive route to performance enhancement, practice is goal-directed repetition of behavior. Although we tend to think of practice as a physical process, it has a mental component as well. Practice leads to proficiency when we train the body to respond with minimal interference from the mind's limbic and sympathetic nervous systems. In mission-critical environments like EMS, it's particularly important that neither emotions nor fight-or-flight instincts impede performance.

Like many of you, I discovered the importance of practice long before I was affiliated with EMS. When I was playing hockey competitively, I needed at least three on-ice sessions a week to subordinate fear of failure (and, as a goaltender, fear of a broken face) to intuition. The stakes aren't as high on a rink as they are in an ambulance, but the need to focus without over-thinking is similar.

We don't often deal with end-of-life events where I work—not a bad thing, considering we're an entertainment complex. Although Kevin and I have a few decades of street experience between us, we rarely ride with that crowd anymore. Consequently, we're challenged daily to prepare for the most difficult scenarios we can imagine, while lacking that extra measure of confidence afforded by daily exposure to complex cases.

Even when I served in busy systems, I didn't feel I was getting enough practice in all the skills I was presumed to have mastered. Cricothyrotomies? The next hole I make in someone's throat will be my first. Intraosseous infusions? Fading memories of forcing stylets into drumsticks limit my inclination to try that on any limbs that don't come with feathers. I knew enough about those procedures to pass my initial exams, but practice in those days was dedicated to memorizing scripts associated with contrived scenarios. It's easier to succeed in test environments where each input is well-defined and leads to a discrete outcome:

Student: *"I administer 1 milligram of Drug A. What do I see?"*

Examiner: *"Your patient becomes unconscious."*

Practice is more important in the field, where our choices and their consequences are almost unlimited. Only by treating real patients do we learn how enigmatic the human body is and how dangerous complacency can be. Without recent hands-on experience, we might as well carry cards with disclaimers like, "Warning: Certification does not guarantee the competence of this individual outside the classroom."

How, then, can we stay current?

Some EMS systems have partnered with local hospitals to offer field providers clinical rotations similar to what's mandated for students. Patient assessment, IV insertion, medication administration, and airway management are examples of procedures that can be monitored by in-house nurses or paramedics. Know your place on the food chain, though. If the attending physician's accountant is invited to try a tube before you are, focus on skills where demand exceeds supply. Let your preceptor know what you hope to accomplish. It helps if you also offer to assist with less glamorous tasks, such as blanket retrieval and bedpan management.

If you work in a system with a volunteer component, donating 5-10 hours a week can supplement your exposure to problematic cases. Already a volunteer? Consider adding to your commitment. The bottom line isn't how much time you contribute; it's how much you can contribute during that time.

Mental simulation is a technique that might help when opportunities for hands-on practice are scarce. Try visualizing a challenging scenario—a cardiac arrest, for example—and then picture the steps you would take to treat your patient. If you have privacy or indulgent partners, you can even go through the motions, literally, of deploying and using your equipment.

Should EMS mandate practice? Some systems do. I needed at least three intubations every six months to keep one job. However, I believe practice, like duty to act, should be driven more by conscientiousness than regulations. We don't care about people only when we're uniformed, and we shouldn't practice only to update our cards. By monitoring and supplementing our clinical experience, we renounce mediocrity as an acceptable standard.

Call it duty to practice.

Author's Note

My remark about intraosseous access is dated, but that doesn't mean I believe sales pitches from drill merchants or reassurance from the AHA that IOs are as benign as peripheral IVs. Let's see what the research says five years from now. Meanwhile, don't mess with my bone marrow.

PARTNERS IN RHYME

2015

I got the first message about Allen at 7:30 on Thanksgiving night. I wasn't surprised my former Opryland partner had lost his battle with a long illness, but I'd hoped his family wouldn't be burdened by a national holiday reminding them of his passing.

It's hard to know what to offer in Allen's memory; so much of what should have been said has been said. I wasn't the only one who thought of Allen as an excellent medic and a good friend. People liked working with him. He was a natural caregiver—someone who didn't need a drug box to help folks feel better.

I wonder if his family knows that.

If it were up to Allen, his kids would be the first priority right now, as always. I'd like to tell them a story I think represents their father's many contributions to patients and partners.

Randy, Teola, and Glen, here's how I met your dad:

We were assigned to work an evening cruise aboard *The General Jackson*. You've probably seen it: a 300-foot showboat with live entertainment and sit-down meals. As usual, we were headed for a three-hour cruise up and down the Cumberland River with a few hundred passengers.

Your father was working his first shift as a paramedic at Opryland. I was there to help him get used to his new job. It usually takes a few months for street medics like your dad to adjust to a fancy place like Opryland.

Your dad and I had barely learned each other's names when we got our first call of the evening: a 45-year-old man who'd had too much to drink and was behaving badly two decks below our office. I quickly explained to your father that this kind of call was a lot like the ones he'd handled except for one special consideration: In the middle of the Cumberland River, EMS is the closest thing to law enforcement. Unless our patient was sick or dangerous enough for us to call 9-1-1, we'd have to babysit him for the rest of the evening.

The guy was from Sweden. He said he loved country music and just wanted to keep drinking while he waited for the show. He kept going back and forth between Swedish and English, which he spoke very well. He smelled like he'd had a lot to drink.

I told him he couldn't have any more alcohol, and suggested we all walk upstairs to our office so your dad and I could check him out. Sometimes when people seem drunk, they're sick with something else. Part of our jobs as paramedics is to consider possibilities like low blood sugar or stroke.

I'm not sure if you saw our office on the boat; it's tiny—just big enough for a cot, a sink, and a couple of cabinets. As soon as the three of us walked in and I shut the door, our patient freaked. He started yelling, "Let me out!" Then he got physical. I was closest to the door, so he tried to go through me. He was younger and a lot bigger. I don't think he wanted to hurt me, but he definitely got my attention.

Your father was there in a second. Instead of fighting with the guy, he was very calm and said, "No problem, just let me get through here." Our patient stopped struggling long enough for your dad to open the door. We stepped outside and went to the port rail, where the big Swede started to cry.

"I'm so sorry," he said, "I was in jail in Sweden. Small rooms scare me."

"No problem," your dad repeated. "We'll hang out here."

"No, it's too late," our patient said. "I just want to die."

He started climbing over the rail. Your dad and I both grabbed him. He wasn't fighting very hard. I think he was more sad than dangerous. Then I had an idea.

"Hey, you said you like country music. How about we sing some?"

At first, the patient seemed surprised, but then he smiled and shouted, "Yes! Good!" Then he started singing "Jackson"; you know, "We got married in a fever . . ." He was pretty good.

Your dad and I let him do Johnny Cash's part; then we came in when it was time for June. It was pretty funny. I don't think the

Opry's going to call us anytime soon, but it did keep him off that rail. The three of us spent the rest of the cruise talking and singing.

Your father must have thought Opryland was a crazy place to work, but he stayed professional and made sure he was never far from me and our patient. That's as safe as I ever felt in EMS.

I'll always remember that call: singing with a suicidal, drunk, Swedish ex-con, and how your dad, on his first day at work, helped make a bad situation better.

I wish I could do the same for you.

MEN AT WORK

2012

To paraphrase Crazy Horse at Little Big Horn, "This is a good day to die"—journalistically speaking. I say that because I mean to write about men and women.

I'm hardly the first to do that. My friend Tracey Loscar authors the marvelous "When Johnny Met Rosie" column for EMS World. It's an essential component of my continuing education. I find the subject matter, women, more rigorous than cardiology and pharmacology combined. If Tracey ever offered certification in AFLS (Advanced Female Listening Skills), I doubt I'd pass without multiple rounds of remediation.

I'm not a newcomer to the topic; you meet lots of women in 59 years. Having spent the last 20 of them in EMS, I can report that fieldwork doesn't shed much light on the subject. Take maternity (please): While the women on scene are reveling in the miracle of birth, I'm thinking, *Wow, that must hurt.*

Even abdominal pain that doesn't yield offspring can be a mystery. I feel woefully unqualified to assess organs that are no more familiar to me than horns or tails . . . I mean wings—no more familiar to me than beautiful, feathery, angelic wings.

Gender-specific perception, rather than physiology, presents the biggest challenge. It's a you're-not-receiving-what-I'm-sending syndrome. I don't understand why that is. Even if women do come from Venus, men come from women. You'd think some of the nurturing propagated by our mothers would penetrate the placental barrier. So why do men other than Alan Alda have trouble showing a sensitive side? Are Y chromosomes blocking our empathy receptors? Is anyone studying that?

A medic who once worked for me expressed similar frustration when we were commiserating about failed efforts at bridging the gender gap with our then-significant others. "Whatever happened to men just being men?" he asked. I didn't know how to answer, mostly because I realized we were . . . gulp . . . sharing our feelings. With each other. In public. It made me want to knit something.

Perhaps men just need better examples set by their role models. Blame *Emergency!* How could we possibly get teary-eyed in front of a guy named Randolph Mantooth? Has there ever been a more alpha-male, in-your-face, don't-touch-my-daughter name than Randolph Mantooth? I doubt it. Now, if Johnny Gage had been played by, say, Lyle Lovett, I think you'd see my male colleagues and me emoting more often.

Men have uses in the field. We lift things. Just this morning, I dragged a 160-pound man from bed. (I wanted to sleep in, but the dogs had to pee.)

We do have strengths beyond strength. I call them the four Ps: protecting, providing, problem-solving, and procreating. At least three of them have everyday uses in EMS:

- We protect partners and patients—sometimes partners from patients, sometimes vice versa.
- We provide life-saving interventions, not to mention serviceable take-out.
- We solve problems directly, emphatically, enthusiastically, and sometimes effectively. That's because we have the ability to focus on therapeutics while ignoring distractors like hidden handguns and toxic waste. My wife, who is also my ex-partner, could tell you stories about my tunnel vision.

Just don't ask us to do more than one of those Ps at a time; we're not good multitaskers. But women are, which begs a not-so-radical recommendation: Why not purposely partner men with women? Wouldn't that cover all the proverbial bases? Empathy would coexist with security in the back of the ambulance as partners played to each other's strengths. And patients of both genders would have access to anatomically correct caregivers. It's a win-win-win-win.

Meanwhile, ladies, there may be hope for me. While I was writing this, I found myself debating The Lovely Helen about the motivations of the characters—not the actors—in a made-for-TV drama I would have termed a chick flick during my less enlightened years. I think

I even used phrases like "Looks aren't everything" and "She thinks she's all that," but only because I've heard Helen say those things about . . . never mind. What's important is, I'm learning. Give me another 10 years and I'll probably cry at *Bambi* sequels.

If you're female and the least bit offended by anything I've said, I apologize—not that I understand why you'd feel that way. But really, I'm sorry for whatever it is I said, or thought about saying, or didn't say, or might at some point in the future think about saying or not saying.

Okay, I'm done. Unlike Custer, I'd rather run than fight.

UNTITLED

A re you a medic or an EMT?
I remember being asked that by an instructor in 1994, soon after I started medic school. It was a rhetorical question. My interrogator was unhappy with my performance during a patient assessment scenario, and seemed eager to stress the differences between EMT-level and paramedic-level skills. I sensed anger and frustration; he was shouting and waving his arms as if his favorite football team had just blown a three-touchdown lead. I'm not a violent person—just ask my cat—but I wanted to hit him. I hollered back, "I'm a medic!" even though that wouldn't be true for another eight months.

I wasn't sure what I was. A hypothetical paramedic? An EMT+? All I know is, I was expected to assert my prospective certification on demand, if not for my benefit then for my instructor's. Hooah.

When I was an EMT, I sometimes felt like a lower life form. It wasn't because of the pay; earning less than medics made sense to me. It was because of chain-of-command assumptions about generic capabilities—communication and decision-making skills—that have less to do with hours spent in classrooms than time on Earth.

I've learned a lot since then: Bench seatbelts won't stop sideways loads, a partner who barks like a Rottweiler will attract the wrong kind of attention, sushi from a diner is riskier than a needle stick, and certification doesn't mean squat about caring or smarts.

The *P* after *EMT* confirms I've demonstrated baseline competence treating synthetic torsos with drugs and electricity during narrated scenarios. It doesn't mean I'm considerate, conscientious, empathetic, or trustworthy. Those qualities—important elements of patient care—have nothing to do with titles.

Classifying caregivers by education or certification means more to EMS providers than to the people we treat. We're very title-conscious in EMS. If I say I'm a medic, my coworkers will know the level of care I'm licensed to deliver. Often, there's a need for that. However, if I introduce myself as a paramedic to outsiders, their conclusions will be much more abstract: *Mike drives an ambulance. Mike sees dead people. Mike will work for less than bartenders make around here.*

I know what I want my patients to think, and it's none of those things. The way I see myself—the way I want people to see me—has less to do with my title than with essential services offered by all levels of field practitioners.

To me, EMS is a noble occupation, independent of title. According to my *Webster's, noble* means "having or showing high moral qualities or ideals, or greatness of character; having excellent qualities." All are important traits for people who take care of others, although "ideals" reminds me we don't always meet those criteria. Hey, even upright posture and opposable thumbs don't make our species perfect, but as long as free will is part of our pedigree, we can do better. Sometimes, EMTs and medics need to remind each other of that.

I'm not too happy with some synonyms for noble: *eminent, lofty, illustrious, grand, stately, splendid, magnificent* and *aristocratic.* Those words imply superiority. I wouldn't want to be that kind of noble. We're supposed to relate to our patients and to each other. That's hard to do in EMS systems with distinct class structure, yet who can deny the prevalence of patient-EMT-medic hierarchies? We should rise above it, or sneak below it, or just ignore it.

My favorite part of our profession is that we provide services of unambiguous value to end-users. No middlemen, just a couple of EMTs with *B, I, P, CC* or *IV* suffixes. I enjoy the innate, title-blind goodness of delivering prehospital care.

Morality, character, excellence—EMS providers at any level can achieve those things. Fulfillment in our industry doesn't depend on titles. Let's rely on each other instead—pool our resources so patients and practitioners benefit from blends of certification and experience.

Next time I'm asked whether I'm a medic or an EMT, I'll answer, "Yes."

A LOYAL
SUBJECT

2014

During my first EMS course, our instructor asked why we wanted to be EMTs. Most of us cited public service as a consideration, but one student—a firefighter in the same district as our classroom—had a different take.

"I just want to be there for my brother firefighters," he said, all but dismissing the possibility of treating people who don't man hoses. I remember thinking there was some value to his sense of loyalty, although I wouldn't qualify for medical care on his watch.

Loyalty is a virtue I prize. When I feel it, I show it without wondering whether it will be reciprocated. Loyalty, like honesty, shouldn't depend on how others think. Once earned, loyalty is a way of saying thanks for being there, and really meaning it.

Here's how I express loyalty:

Not talking behind your back. When you're the topic of conversation in absentia, I'll make sure you have at least one ally.

Preferential treatment. I'll pass along opportunities that might interest you.

Responding to emergencies. I'll do my best to answer up when you need me.

The open-fly provision. When there's a clear and present danger of indignity, I'll let you know as delicately as possible.

Some people are more attuned to communal loyalty; a Red Sox fan, for example—not a bad thing to be since last October, but much less committed than the kind of loyalty I'm talking about. When I feel loyalty, I want to give back—to help as I was helped. Sports fans and their teams don't owe each other anything.

Loyalty to EMS sounds as superficial to me as any other institutional allegiance. It's hard for me to feel loyal to an industry. Consider the well-meaning provider who credits EMS for professional development. That's a nice sentiment, but hard to support with gestures of loyalty. Perhaps I'm missing a spiritual connection or two.

Do I owe EMS? I've thought about that a lot since leaving the field. My life was more interesting and less predictable on ambulances than in offices. The daily challenges of patient care raised the stakes of problem-solving; the highs were higher and the lows lower. Corporate life—an occupational endpoint my high-school classmates and I were hard-wired to chase—turned out to be tedious compared to patient care. I'm glad I discovered that 22 years ago, before committing to another two decades of desktop decision-making.

Those big, boring businesses where I got my start paid pretty well, though, and allowed me to raise a family-and-a-half with much less struggle than I would have faced as a 21-year-old paramedic. I haven't thought much about the gap between my theoretical and actual earnings—until now. Let's just say whatever I might have owed EMS for a ticket to the urban version of Mr. Toad's Wild Ride has been paid in full.

I feel loyalty to people, not organizations. In EMS, that means:

Partners. It's hard to overstate the importance of compatible coworkers. When pairings click, there's a sense of shared proficiency greater than the sum of individual skills. There's also fundamental trust that makes it easier to confront unknown aspects of every scene. More than once, partners compensated for my inadequate situational awareness. It's hard not to feel loyal to people who help you get home safely.

Instructors. The best teachers don't limit their availability to classrooms or office hours. I remember frantic phone calls I made to instructors who knew the difference between bad students and bad days. Those who went beyond the curriculum to answer questions and offer assistance earned my loyalty.

Employers. I never signed a contract, but I always felt my employers and I had an understanding: As long as I was conscientious and competent, my boss would provide the salary and benefits promised when I was hired. That might not sound special, but 40 years of working for others convinced me that in the workplace, chronic fairness is rare and worthy of loyalty.

There's a fourth group very much an object of my loyalty: you, our readers. You didn't have to browse this magazine and you didn't have to turn to this page. Thank you for doing so. I promise I'll keep trying to deliver content that meets your standards. It's a matter of loyalty.

Author's Note

I wrote that last paragraph when Life Support was a monthly magazine column. "Our readers" are now my readers. I thank you all for your loyalty.

PACK
MENTALITY

2010

In my household, it's tempting to measure the passage of time in dog years. Maybe that's because my wife and I are outnumbered by four-legged companions: two dogs plus a cat who thinks he's a cocker spaniel. For those of you not certified in ACLS (Approximate Canine Life Span), one dog year averages seven human years of existence. That's a lot of living crammed into 12 months; hence the expression "party animal."

I'm only eight canine years old. I didn't get started in EMS until I was, let's see, 5½—a lot later than most. While you old dogs were rotating tourniquets and transmitting telemetry from small suitcases, I was into my second decade (my first "dog-cade") as a corporate carnivore. This was in the '80s, when a whole genre of business books tried to distill profitability into a few buzzwords. Most of those works were of less consequence than the average music video, but one book that still engenders almost biblical reverence is *In Search of Excellence* by Tom Peters and Bob Waterman. Although my copy is looking a little jaundiced, its content is as relevant and thought-provoking as it was when Rex—I mean Reagan—was in the White House.

I retreated to my bookshelf this morning because I've been preoccupied with the future of our industry. I blame my colleague, Skip Kirkwood, who has a knack for raising significant issues, such as enhanced education, quality of care, and compensation. Recently, Skip tackled EMS inertia—our tendency to resist change even when there's evidence some of our practices are ineffective and obsolete. Part of the problem is parochialism—regional chauvinism that subordinates global imperatives to local customs. I agree with Skip that "courageous leadership" is needed to infuse EMS with something more than personal preferences and anecdotes. *In Search of Excellence* is a robust resource worth examining.

The essence of the book is the authors' claim that they discovered eight characteristics common to well-managed companies. Seven are relevant to EMS:

A bias for action. As emergent care providers, we're trained to act. *Do something* rivals *Do no harm* as a prehospital imperative. Some of us lose that proactive predisposition when we acquire supervisory responsibilities. Are we too worried about political correctness and executive backlash to try new solutions for old problems? Who among us will dare to be different?

Close to the customer. Most EMS providers know not to let long hours and low pay interfere with good medicine. Are we equally uncompromising about patient advocacy? When we allow some citizens' system abuses to foster an us-against-them attitude, we tarnish not only our own reputations, but also the public's perception of our profession.

Autonomy and entrepreneurship. Street medicine offers more autonomy than most occupations. Providers who require lots of handholding probably should consider other careers. Entrepreneurship, uncommon at EMS's administrative levels, is much more prevalent among the rank and file, many of whom rely on multiple revenue-producing activities to pay bills. Smart managers nurture new ideas and encourage innovation, regardless of the source.

Productivity through people. Leadership isn't about organizing gripe sessions and group hugs; it means giving workers the tools to succeed, then expecting them to do so. Delegating responsibility is part of the process, but employees also need feedback about corporate objectives and control over their areas of accountability. The headline from management should be "I trust you," not "I like you."

Hands-on, value driven. Talking about values is easy; instilling them is hard work. Good examples must be set from the top down. If your boss preaches safety, then assigns you and your partner to a rig with paroxysmal electronics, the message is "Everyone for themselves."

Simple form, lean staff. This tenet is about decoupling complexity from growth. As companies expand, practical limitations to each administrator's scope of responsibility dictate new reporting relationships. Decentralization and flexible, user-friendly systems can minimize layers of management and facilitate bidirectional flow of timely information. However, we must guard against unrealistic corporate expectations that often accompany indiscriminate paring of staff.

Simultaneous loose-tight properties. Even a decentralized organization with lots of low-level empowerment needs ongoing reinforcement of core values from above. It's like reminding our kids of their curfews before they borrow our cars.

The theme of *In Search of Excellence* is clear: Simple practices based on devotion to customers (i.e., patients) and respect for employees lead to successful ventures. That sounds easy to execute. It's not. There's a shortage of experienced EMS supervisors with the requisite traits—selflessness, passion for quality, and big-picture awareness—to promote organizational excellence. We can look to our non-exempt ranks for tomorrow's champions, but the stars we seek are not necessarily high-profile clinicians. And management courses are not yet part of mainstream paramedic curricula.

Must we import our next generation of leaders from other industries? I don't think so. If you alpha males and females who've already implemented excellence at regional levels share a few of your best of breed with the rest of us, they'll find plenty of opportunities to apply your teachings in new and challenging environments. Meanwhile, you'll backfill with other young pups who want to be pack leaders someday. Sounds like a win tin tin.

Enough with the dog metaphor. It's time for my walk.

Author's Note

We're up to two dogs and three cats, only one of which was with us in 2010. They are equally excellent.

STRONG WORK

2014

I'm not much of a singer, but I do it anyway—mostly in the car, and only when the closest amateur music critic is at least a bus length ahead or behind.

I sing in the key of Frog. The Lovely Helen calls the effect disturbing. Well, we can't all be The King, or even Prince. Knowing our limitations is an important part of good citizenship. Often, the best we can do is play to our strengths while encouraging others to do the same.

When I helped produce a CD of EMS-themed songs last year, there was no doubt my value, if any, to the project would be administrative: budgeting, scheduling, packaging, marketing, and sales—not very exciting, but as essential to the music business as documentation is to EMS.

Working on that CD reminded me it's okay not to be good at everything. EMS allows for that. I've never seen a policy, protocol, algorithm, or curriculum that assumed practitioners apply impeccable reason in the realm of all things possible. Much of our prehospital guidance is in the form of easy-to-process bullet points which are intended to buffer crew members' fallible memory. And when written rules aren't flexible enough, there's always medical control—an often-undervalued reservoir of good advice.

Knowing how and when to get help is just as important as the advice itself. Unless you and your partner routinely share ideas with Solomon-like propriety, there will be calls when one of you doesn't make the best use of the other. Can the two of you talk about that? Competition, insecurity, and ego sometimes make it hard to offset weaknesses with pooled strengths.

Early in my career, I rode with a medic who insisted on doing all of our airway management. Sometimes he'd apologize by explaining he considered intubation "a manhood thing." Lucky for me I had plenty of FTOs who didn't feel that way.

During primary training, when habits are works in progress, it's important to understand the connection between strengths and preferences. Strengths often become preferences (and vice versa), but over-indulging the latter can hinder development of the former. Forcing ourselves to engage in less-comfortable tasks can expand our capabilities. We just have to guard against thinking of our patients as manikins. Unwavering determination to succeed is admirable when running a marathon; not so much when puncturing a patient.

There were times in the field I said, or perhaps only thought, "Just one more try" when a coworker might have been more successful. All of us need practice, but we have to recognize when someone else's talent is a better match for the emergency of the moment. There's more at stake than bragging rights; most importantly, a favorable outcome.

Sometimes, EMS mixes its message to caregivers by simultaneously lauding individualism and teamwork, as if decisiveness were a trait partners should employ separately yet concurrently. I don't know about you, but I've rarely seen that work. Someone needs to recognize when weaknesses compound, rather than offset. Even with two alpha medics, at least one had better be willing to take direction.

In the field, I never felt I had a monopoly on insight. I learned, as a new medic, to value contributions from every crewmember regardless of certification. I still believe authority is something you titrate when, despite your best intentions, teamwork isn't yielding a critical next step. Reviewing those moments as a group decreases the chances they'll be repeated.

The most capable people I know are also the ones who most readily admit their faults. They seem to see their talents as gifts, rather than as rewards or rights. I think they try to leverage strengths like the rest of us, but they have better timing; they can spot opportunities for collaboration from a distance and feel energized—not threatened—by the prospect of mutual success. They know being strong means sharing strengths while acknowledging weaknesses.

I'm no singer. Then again, Elvis was no EMT.

Author's Note

I've been fascinated by music since childhood, when my parents paid for clarinet, saxophone, and oboe lessons. I think I would have done better with a more popular instrument—drums, perhaps, or a guitar. Now I mess around with one of those electronic keyboards. The technology is impressive; my talent is not.

SHOULD I STAY OR SHOULD I GO?

2016

For many of us, EMS is the second-hardest thing we'll do. Even more difficult—and I'm speaking from personal experience—is *leaving* EMS.

It was a struggle for me to start a new career as a paramedic at 41. I had doubts all the way through school, but I stayed optimistic about making a difference in the human condition—not much of a possibility when I was manufacturing cosmetics for a living.

Although I wasn't a natural caregiver, EMS turned out to be a good fit. It was a chance to apply my engineering background to a whole new discipline: medicine. Years before I left, I knew I'd miss it. I tried to remind myself of that whenever I'd get frustrated by calls or employers or rules. When I finally quit 9-1-1 for good in 2013, I felt I'd gotten enough out of it to leave with good memories and no regrets.

I was wrong about the regrets part. I still second-guess myself about resigning and torment my sainted wife with on-again, off-again plans to return. Then, logic—usually hers—prevails and I stay retired.

My decision to leave EMS had been sudden and simple: After recovering from another back injury, I was treating an unstable cardiac patient when I realized I couldn't rely on my legs for kneeling or lifting. I quit the same day.

Most of you won't have such an easy choice. You'll agonize over the pros and cons of the job for months or even years. Some of you shouldn't wait that long, because symptoms of a career in crisis are already compromising your performance and quality of life:

You dread going to work. Maybe EMS isn't for you. There's no shame in admitting a wrong turn on your career path. Change course and find something you enjoy. I've done that five times in 45 years.

It hurts too much physically. EMS requires strength and agility. When pain prevents you from bending or lifting, you're a potential liability to your partners. Don't wait for them to notice. If the problem can't be fixed, leave on your own terms.

It hurts too much mentally. Some colleagues speak of burn-out as a temporary condition that gets resolved after a few weeks of doing something else. I disagree. You might hate your job less for a few months, but the same dissatisfiers will still be there, waiting for triggers. Burnt-out medics are risks to themselves and everyone around them.

Patients have become a nuisance. Consider this recent Facebook post from a paramedic: "Manual (CPR) may be better, but I have no intention of providing quality CPR like I did when I was twenty. Now I'm apt to do a good 2 minutes' worth and call it for physical exhaustion or spite." If patients make you feel that way—spiteful, vengeful, resentful, inconvenienced, or angry—do yourself and them a favor: Walk away from EMS.

You've fallen far behind the knowledge curve. Mandatory CME merely reminds us what we should already know. Learning new material is up to us. Keeping up with the science of medicine is a job within the job.

The risks clearly outweigh the benefits. EMS has come a long way in identifying threats to providers: blood-borne pathogens, unsafe lifting, work-related violence, and PTSD, for example. Even as those dangers and others are addressed, there will always be above-average odds of illness and injury. Look elsewhere if you're seeking a risk-free profession.

You're hurting your family. Do you find EMS so unpleasant, you routinely act out your frustrations in front of your family? Occasional venting to a significant other might be therapeutic, but chronic impatience, anger, or worse can victimize those closest to you and leave you without a support system when you need it most.

You suffer from unrelenting anxiety. A little nervousness in the field helps us focus and reminds us we're engaged in a serious business. Overwhelming anxiety is another matter; it can interfere with performance and make sufferers non-functional. If you struggle to keep your composure on calls, consider a change.

You've lost hope of making things better. The possibility of making a difference attracts many of us to EMS. We acquire more realistic views of our limitations over time, but I think most of us continue to feel like rescuers even if we don't have many opportunities to show it.

During my 20 years in the field, I wasn't the most experienced or best-qualified responder, but I always wanted to be the one answering the toughest calls. I liked the challenge of overcoming obstacles to do what was expected of me. I don't think I'll ever stop feeling that way.

Find a job you know you'll miss, then do it as long as you can.

THE ESSENCE OF EMS

2016

Larry Zacarese isn't home nearly as much as he'd like to be. The assistant police chief and director of emergency management at Stony Brook University in New York is also a paramedic and attorney, either of which could limit his discretionary time to, say, weekend mornings before sunrise. When Larry's wife, Yvonne, asks him about his workday, I'm guessing she's already cleared her schedule for at least the next 30 minutes.

It's a vibrant life, but not one Larry had imagined when I met him in medic school 22 years ago. He wanted to be a cop like his dad, uncle, and great-uncle. New York City was the biggest, most messed-up place he could do that east of the Mississippi—perfect for Larry, who wasn't raised to take anything easy.

Zacarese got his wish in 1998: He graduated NYPD's academy and was assigned to the 113th precinct in Jamaica, Queens—not known for its serenity. Larry embraced his beat as the proving ground it was, and tried not to lose all hope for humanity when the viciousness of the streets exhausted the patience of both cops and paramedics.

On the morning of September 11th, 2001, Zacarese started a vacation that lasted only until the first jetliner hit the first 110-story tower. Larry's life, like so many others, changed forever in an instant. He told his dad he wasn't coming home until the rescuing was done. None of us knew it already was.

After a few days, saving turned to salvage at Ground Zero. Officer Zacarese worked at the world's biggest crime scene for another three months because that's what he was told to do.

The following summer, toward the end of a four-month training program for the city's elite Emergency Services Unit (ESU), Larry started having trouble catching his breath. His persistent cough and low peak-flow readings disqualified him for the scuba component of ESU. He transferred to K-9 and completed their requisite schooling in six weeks, using an inhaler as a hedge against his newly diagnosed reactive airway disease.

By 2004, Zacarese was tired all the time. His list of prescribed medications resembled the formulary of a 60-year-old COPDer. He was promoted to sergeant and stayed with NYPD until the Stony Brook position opened in 2009—well short of the 20+ years he'd planned in the city. Regret isn't what he feels, though.

"Mostly I'm pissed," the 40-year-old Long Island native says. "I'm angry about what happened to the country, what happened to my friends, and what's continuing to happen to them. Every day they're either battling to stay alive or dying. After 15 years, it's only getting worse.

"I've never wished I didn't go. I've never said, 'Why did this happen to me?' I'm just pissed off it happened at all."

A source of frustration is the assurances Larry and his WTC co-workers got about safety from desk-bound officials who should have known better.

"We went with the advice we were given," Zacarese says. "People tell you, 'The air's safe.' Bullshit. A block away, it was still death and destruction—acrid smoke and bodies. It's not like they misjudged; they knew. Here we are 15 years later and people who were there are sick and dying or already dead."

Larry hopes EMS is better equipped to resolve what he considers the No. 1 operational deficiency during 9/11: communications. "We still see those problems whenever we drill. You have to be able to talk to each other, listen to each other, and follow commands."

The father of four tries to educate the uninitiated about what to expect when the next disaster hits, but such advice, even when backed by hard-earned experience, isn't always popular.

"Part of the problem today is that a lot of our new people were very young when 9/11 happened. For them, it's ancient history. It's like trying to get someone my age to understand Vietnam. I was just a kid during that war. I'm not going to be able to relate to the veterans who lived through that.

"For me as a cop and a medic, 9/11 was a defining moment. I know lots of others who responded and feel the same. If it happened again, I'd kiss my wife and kids and I'd go, because that's what we do. It sounds like some corny movie line, but that's what I believe."

★★★

Rob DeMeo, 37, is a paramedic for MedicOne Medical Response in Nashville, Tennessee. That's a long way from Huntington, New York, where Rob was born, and from West Street in Manhattan, where he was staged with Hunter Ambulance between 1 and 2 World Trade Center on the morning of 9/11/2001.

"I was thinking we should have helmets like the FDNY guys, because debris was falling all around us," DeMeo recalls. "No one thinks about private ambulances needing helmets.

"The debris started getting bigger—computer components and insulation, then steel. It made a lot of noise falling from that height, but I didn't see anyone get hit. Then I heard some guy scream, 'Everybody run!'

"There was a rushing sound like another airplane, so I turned away from the building and started running. When I saw a debris cloud in front of me, I knew it wasn't a plane; I just assumed the top of the tower had fallen off.

"I was caught between the building and the cloud. I just covered myself and kept running. I wasn't thinking about dying. At 22, that doesn't seem possible. I just didn't want it to hurt."

Rob suffered a broken leg, a head laceration, and burns to his back. He was triaged in Manhattan, then transferred to a hospital on Long Island. He says he's fully recovered and has no regrets.

"I don't think I was there long enough to be bummed out about it, or as scarred as the people who were there longer. My on-scene time was probably two hours tops—not enough to leave a lasting impact.

"It's like a dream that gets harder and harder to remember. Sometimes I feel like, was I really there?"

DeMeo became a paramedic two years later and joined Delaware's New Castle County system. He relocated to Nashville in 2008, where he's continued to work in EMS. He says he doesn't think much about 9/11 until he hears about other terrorist incidents.

"I think I know what some of those victims go through—the confusion, the feeling of being lost. On 9/11, the street corner I'd been standing on became unrecognizable. I couldn't even tell which direction to walk."

In the aftermath of an attack, it's normal to want to assign responsibility, but Rob thinks conspiracy theories are weakened by people who try too hard to force a fit. "It's like blaming somebody other than the Japanese for Pearl Harbor," he says. "I'm not sure why our culture and our education system can't simply accept that the people who hijacked those planes are the ones responsible."

Educating people about 9/11 is something DeMeo knows he can do. It can be hard, though, to accommodate the opinions of those who were somewhere else that day.

"I'd rather just listen to others act like experts about it, and not even let them know I was there. I've learned to get entertainment value from them instead of feeling angry.

"What I think is most important to take away from that day is how our jobs and our lives can change in a fraction of a second."

★★★

The last time I wrote about 9/11 was five years ago; I did a column about Larry in 2011 and one about Rob in 2009. Checking in with them seemed like a good way to start a story about the 15th anniversary of that day.

Both medics downplayed the personal consequences of their service. They spoke more of healing than hurting, and denied having second thoughts about participating in their nation's most lethal MCI.

I sensed they omitted their most disturbing memories, perhaps because there are no words to describe such things to those who weren't there. More importantly, they had no trouble articulating the essence of EMS: not heroic rescue, but simply being bold and sharp when weeks of tedium become moments of terror.

I think EMS has changed a lot in the last 15 years. We're focusing more on chronic illness and well care while acquiring new technology to better diagnose acute conditions like STEMI and sepsis. To me, we seem like an occupation in search of a role.

Maybe we're looking too hard. Maybe we need responders like Zacarese and DeMeo to remind us that our primary mission is to show up when others can't or won't. I have a feeling we're going to be needing lots of that.

Author's Note

The 15ᵗʰ anniversary of 9/11 was the last time I wrote about that subject. I felt I'd said everything worth saying by someone who didn't work at Ground Zero until a week after the towers fell. I think it's important to honor WTC responders like Larry and Rob without implying that an EMT or paramedic card, alone, links one spiritually to the first-person spectacle of that day. Those who were there know what the rest of us can't.

LOST IN TRANSLATION

2013

As I was channel-surfing in a restful state shortly after last Christmas, I happened upon a Monty Python marathon. Such instances of good fortune are why I label myself an optimist.

I freakin' love Monty Python. The British comedy troupe skewered '70s society with iconoclastic parodies as clever as they were absurd. If being a Python had been a career choice, I never would have finished engineering school.

It would be difficult for a Python fan (Pythonite? Pythian?) to pick a favorite sketch, but I don't think any were funnier than the Hungarian phrasebook bit: A Hungarian tourist walks into a London smoke shop wanting to buy cigarettes. After consulting his flawed Hungarian-English dictionary, he tells the tobacconist, "I will not buy this record, it is scratched." When the clerk looks perplexed, the tourist scans his booklet again, then adds "My hovercraft is full of eels." The scene degenerates into a fistfight when the Hungarian inadvertently antagonizes a police officer with "You have beautiful thighs."

I don't remember any of my futile attempts at street Spanish leading to violence, but I've worked many calls where patients and I have become frustrated at our inability to communicate. I think some non-English speakers assumed I was being obstinate when all I was trying to do was understand their complaints—not a radical way of beginning care.

One source of help is translation services that promise to connect customers to native speakers of almost any language within seconds of phoned-in requests. Not a bad idea, but when I simulated a call from the field, I found the interpreter on the line wasn't comfortable with medical terms like *seizures* or *anti-depressant*. And then there's the matter of involving a third party in a confidential discussion. Gaining consent would be easier if there weren't a language barrier in the first place.

I'm thinking the solution might be as close as our smartphones. You do have one, don't you? Sorry, I don't mean to sound obnoxious. Being an early adapter of the latest technology is a new experience for me. Now that I've signed up for more data per month than I've stored, cumulatively, on every PC I've ever owned, I've been looking for apps that enhance my productivity instead of my pastimes.

One is called Translate. It works just the way you'd expect: Type a word or phrase in one language, see or hear a translation in another. I decided to test that app with a slightly idiomatic English phrase before progressing to something medical; I entered *I want to see how well this whole translation thing works* and requested Spanish, the second most popular language in the world (per About.com) and second most common language spoken around here. Here's what Translate gave me: *Quiero ver lo bien que funciona todo esto de la traducción.*

It works, I thought. Then I remembered I don't speak Spanish well enough to know that, so I put the exact Spanish phrase back into the translator and asked for English. I got *I want to see how well this works in translation.* Close, but not the same intent I'd expressed idiomatically. I wasn't surprised Translate didn't digitize verbal subtleties accurately. That would have been a lot to expect of a device that still can't process body language.

Next, I wondered if I could rely on Translate to interpret basic medical questions—the kind we ask patients during every assessment. I chose a common question—*What does the pain feel like?*—and requested translations into each of the world's ten most popular languages (other than English). Here's what I got when I converted those foreign phrases back into English:

Chinese (Mandarin): *Feeling of pain is what?*

Spanish: *What is pain?*

Arabic: *Why the pain feel like?*

Hindi: *What kind of pain do you think?*

Portuguese: *What does the pain feel like?*

Bengali: *What is pain?*

Russian: *What does the pain feel like?*

Japanese: *What pain I would feel?*

German: *What does the pain feel like?*

Four (Chinese, Spanish, Bengali, and Arabic) were more philosophical than clinical, the Hindi translation sounded adversarial, and Japanese was just plain weird. Only the Portuguese, Russian, and German translations were precise.

The Translate app is impressive; it's compact, free, easy to use, and not terribly inaccurate. I see it inspiring a new prehospital caveat, though: Treat the patient, not the smartphone.

Author's Note

Eight years later, translation apps are a lot more popular. I use mine all the time, mostly so I can follow The Godfather in the original Sicilian.

SOX EDUCATION

2014

You're probably expecting something about EMS in this space. We'll get to that. First, let's talk about sox, or socks, if you're not a fan of Red or White. I'm sporting a pair of brown ones right now because socks are something I was taught to wear even on steamy summer days, when they're about as welcome as toques. (Memo to readers in southern North America: A toque is a Canadian sock for the head. My friend, Sandy, from Ontario assures me Canadians also wear socks on their feet.)

The Lovely Helen and I disagree on the importance of fresh socks. She complains I monopolize our washing machine, not to mention her discretionary time, by changing my socks daily. "Did you just dump your whole sock drawer into the laundry?" she's been known to ask. So I've been thinking, maybe I don't have to change my socks every day just because I've always done so. Perhaps slavish devotion to custom doesn't produce the best outcomes.

I've heard medics characterize their jobs as routine. They say they diagnose patients from doorways, treat, transport, and never look back. They tell me their ambulances are extensions of ERs; that the biggest difference between doctors and paramedics is income. They pride themselves on their independence—tolerating, but not needing, oversight. I say these are signs of apathy, not expertise.

Yet I so wanted to be that kind of unperturbable medic. I imagined arriving on scene with nothing more than a penlight, sensing sickness behind my patient's rheumy eyes, then declaring "pneumonia" while awestruck junior crew members merely confirmed my diagnosis with their clumsy analytics. Oh, the inevitability of it all.

I assumed the path to paramedic omnipotence began with mastery of the curriculum. If a disease had a protocol, I was all over it. That ruled in the classroom; not so much in the field. As I look back on my earliest mistakes, I think most of them were caused by lack of imagination. I was determined to fit presenting problems into contrived cases that ended as predictably as they'd begun. Rigid adherence to hypotheticals didn't leave room for the variability of real-world conditions, such as multiple complaints and causes.

Knowing when not to act is as important as mastering any treatment algorithm. In *Taigman's Advanced Cardiology*, the author recounts the making of a "cardiac cripple" through needless, protocol-driven administration of bradycardia meds. Contrary to classroom imperatives, parroting "atropine" for heart rates below 60 can be more dangerous than doing nothing at all.

My wife survived an instance of such cookbook medicine when she was hospitalized last summer. For Helen, being in a hospital is like me being on a roller coaster: terror tempered by hysteria. The only thing she hates more than hospitals is . . . I can't think of anything. As she was awaiting discharge—anxious and in pain—after major surgery, a physician noticed her blood pressure was up. Ya think? The attending told Helen hospital rules required her to stay until her BP came down, and ordered Lopressor.

Helen was panicky when she called me to rescue her. I broke laws driving to that hospital. I bet I would have qualified for Lopressor, too.

My wife needed peace of mind, not beta blockers. Any policy that said otherwise clearly was inappropriate. To blithely follow such directives is neither efficient nor therapeutic; it's foolish. I think any medical professional who allows habit and complacency to override common sense should find another line of work.

I think most of us find a middle ground between anarchy and doing everything by the book. At an organizational level, that means a willingness to adopt policies that would have been labeled heresy two decades ago, like BLS Narcan, limited O_2, and delayed intubation. No one expects EMS agencies to invent the next standard of care; just follow the latest evidentiary wisdom before books are written about it.

Individual providers are certified to exercise judgment by keeping current on the potential consequences of bad decisions. Biennial or triennial expiration dates acknowledge the role of new research in shaping prehospital practices. I'm afraid caregivers who scoff at refreshers and other continuing education as timewasters, and who feel experience alone should be a ticket to recertification, will be last to recognize flawed methods.

It's summer in Nashville. Should be a good day to go without socks.

SEEING IS BELIEVING

2012

It's not always busy where I work. Let me rephrase that: I'm rarely busy, at least not in the conventional paramedic sense of busyness.

If you were to count the number of employees, performers, and guests needing medical assistance at Opryland, most days you wouldn't have enough to justify both Johnny and Roy standing by. A perpetual shortage of sick people at our entertainment complex leaves me with discretionary time that many of you don't have. I could run serial 12 leads on myself, or sort syringes by lot number, or help my non-medical coworkers dispense customer service imaginatively and emphatically with therapeutic doses of southern hospitality. I routinely choose the latter, which is how I became Minister of Elevator Operations on *The General Jackson*, Opryland's 300-foot showboat.

In December, while I was helpfully transporting guests two decks down from the boarding area in the aft lift, one of them commented that I must have the best job in the world. I hear this a lot—something about being paid to work on a boat on a lazy river on a nice day. It's easier to just nod and grin than describe the healthcare issues I face whenever the spit hits the fantail. On this day, I said, "Well, the real challenge is staying prepared," or something equally pithy. A passenger replied, "You mean in case it breaks?"

The elevator. He meant the elevator. You see, we don't wear EMS patches at Opryland. Except for the scissors sticking out of my pants pocket, there were no visual cues to contradict his assumption that elevators are my life. (Do they use trauma shears to fix those things?) The doors opened before I had a chance to explain.

Afterward, I had mixed feelings about the encounter. I don't mind helping wherever I'm needed, and I appreciated the humor of the moment, but I'm proud of my real job, too. I would have liked to persuade my captive audience that downtime in the essential services isn't time off—it's time between emergencies, and making use of that time while maintaining readiness is a skill in itself.

Preconceived notions were my chief constraint. Even if I'd been outfitted in state-of-the-art buff stuff, my passengers' opinions of me—and probably of EMS—would have depended more on delivering them to the right floors than on anything I could have preached about prehospital care.

Part of the problem is that EMS's backstory—training, anticipation, and a willingness to engage—isn't nearly as interesting as the exaggerated images of lifesaving choreographed for prime-time TV. And people experiencing real emergencies are too preoccupied with survival to appreciate the subtleties of our work. Other than the most stirring street-side resuscitations, I think our best opportunities to enhance public perception of EMS come between calls, when impressionable bystanders are relaxed and more receptive.

I've written about downtime before, but only from an in-house perspective. Not all of our downtime is staged at headquarters. Consider the public's perception of these very visible, on-duty pastimes:

Eating. Unless you and your partner routinely order in, someone has to venture outside to gather consumables for the coming shift. No problem but not everyone watching will sympathize if the need to feed becomes an extended sit-down meal at Budget Burger, accompanied by animated shop talk.

Sleeping. You know you're getting acclimated to EMS when sleep is mediated more by opportunity than by need. However, if the moment strikes while you're riding shotgun on the way back from the hospital, in full view of pedestrians at each red light, don't be surprised if you're the subject of a sarcastic YouTube video entitled, "EMS Hard at Work."

Shopping. Some of my employers allowed us to run personal errands between calls. Window-gazing at the local mega-mall was a stress-reliever—for us, not for our fellow shoppers. Our mere presence at public facilities prompts two questions from onlookers: *Is there an emergency?* and *Shouldn't you be responding to one?*

Smoking. Yes, it's unfair you can't smoke when it doesn't bother someone else. Yes, it will always bother someone else.

I'm adding EMT (elevator management technician) to my personal list of downtime imperatives. Barring free fall or premature rupture of membranes, I doubt I'll have a chance to prove my true worth between floors. I'll just try to be the best vertical transport medic east of Station 51.

Going up.

Author's Note

At various times, Opryland patrons also assumed I was an usher, a waiter, a lifeguard, an athletic trainer, and an exterminator. All fit my employer's expanded scope of paramedic practice except exterminator.

THIS IS A TEST

2010

I hate taking tests. I'm using the word *hate* because *dislike* isn't strong enough. I dislike snow, cold soup, movies with subtitles, and teams that beat the Red Sox, but I don't hate them (well, maybe the Yankees a little bit). None of them aggravate me as much as EMS exams. Oral, practical, written—I dread them all. I'm afraid I'll forget the year Napoleon dispatched the first ambulance; or I won't verbalize donning a full body condom to treat a spider bite. My memory's not what it used to be. I still can't believe I learned New York City's protocols before I knew a platelet from a placenta.

I suppose we have it easier than some professions. Bar exams in most states last two days. London taxi drivers are tested on 300 routes covering 25,000 streets. That's roughly four times the combined number of bones, muscles, joints, ligaments, and tendons in the human body. Next time I'm in London, I'm doing a ride-along with a cabbie instead of a medic.

As a student in the early 1970s, I had a casual attitude about exams. I was so apathetic, I came this close (picture Mike's thumb and forefinger spread the width of an EpiPen) to spending the last two years of college at the racetrack. I wasn't setting very challenging goals for myself. I'd decided any grade-point average that didn't rule out a cap and gown was acceptable. More than once, my pre-med roommates were astonished at my cavalier acceptance of C's and D's. "I passed, didn't I?" was my mantra. I blamed the capitalist, imperialist, military/industrial complex for my indifference. Or maybe it was Woodstock.

Then, as Dr. Seuss might say, something went bump. I started to take pride in scholarship. I wish I could tell you I awoke one morning with a hunger for knowledge, but I was driven more by competition, and maybe a milliequivalent of resentment. It felt good to do almost as well as those brainiacs with pocket protectors and arthritic personalities. By the end of my senior year, I'd accumulated enough A's and B's to graduate *cum mediocritas* with a 2.8 GPA—sufficient to assure prospective employers I could use a slide rule, at least. I climbed the corporate hierarchy without having to recite scripted industrial scenarios like, "You arrive at the assembly line to find two employees who want to take bathroom breaks at the same time..."

I became exam-averse two decades and four careers later in medic school, on the Thursday before the Tuesday when we were beginning ALS ambulance rotations in New York City. I had passed that week's written test and was competing with classmates for slots at practical stations that would certify me as Less Ignorant Than Last Week or relegate me to another round of remediation. My final assignment was to start an IV and a dopamine drip on one of those vinyl arms with veins the size of water mains. I remember narrating my interventions as I'd been taught—confidently and methodically—to my preceptor, Scott, whom I would one day work with.

I scarcely noticed the minutes passing. Scott did, perhaps because there were so many of them. At the end of the drill, during which the sun set in more than one time zone, Scott politely informed me that while I had been diligent in performing each step of the scenario, an actual patient would have long since succumbed—to old age, not shock. He did praise my enunciation, though.

Until then, I hadn't failed an EMS exam. I was angry and embarrassed. Scared, too, because I'd just blown the first of only two chances to pass that station. I wanted to do it again—*now*—but there would be no retests until the following week. It was a long four days until I demonstrated more timely delivery of emergent medication.

That experience cemented my austere outlook on test-taking:

We're only as good as our last performance. Each time we're evaluated is a fresh opportunity to screw up. There's no extra credit for prior achievement. Just because I can intubate a manikin from across the room doesn't mean I know what a pancreas is.

Evaluating practical exams is a subjective exercise. I was relieved to pass my second IV infusion attempt, but I might not have with a different preceptor. What if the examiner administering my retest counted 40 drops per minute instead of 30, or decided my technique wasn't sufficiently sterile? At what point should instructors derail students' careers by dealing the "automatic failure" card?

Passing is not enough. Even after overcoming my initial awkwardness at the IV station, I was still uneasy about doing drips in prime time. Written exams were hardly confidence builders, either. Scoring 80 when 75 earned you a card was no reason to celebrate; it was motivation to master the remaining 20%.

We test the science, not the art. I think most EMS providers would agree they've learned much more in the field than in the classroom. The challenge is how to quantify and evaluate intuition. Should EMS practical exams consist of monitored field exercises rather than contrived scripts?

Two months after graduation, I joined the faculty. It was strange to be on the other side of the desk. I tried to balance students' aspirations and the safety of their future patients. When candidates' failures triggered tears, excuses, or pleas for second chances, I was reminded of how harsh the testing environment can be. It's a grueling process for examiners and examinees, with no video replay to validate close calls. I'm sure I didn't always get those right.

Soon it will be time for me to reestablish my own competence. Let's see, 1973: federal funding of EMS. Or was that the debut of *Emergency!*?

OUT OF SERVICE

2013

Two decades before I earned my first EMS paycheck, I manufactured cosmetics for a living. If that sounds glamorous to you, I can't even imagine what kind of day you must be having.

My prime directive for most of those years was to ensure quality while minimizing costs—typical responsibilities for bosses in industrial environments. Service was a priority, too—well, sort of. We had no direct contact with retail customers. We assumed they were out there because if they weren't, we reasoned, none of us would have jobs. Our only contribution to customer service was to keep our warehouses stocked with every conceivable shade of feel-good products so the pharmacy next to the hardware store on Main Street would have enough Lip Tenderizer to make Mrs. Brown's daughter lovely on Saturday night.

Even if you're new to EMS, you're probably much more directly involved in customer service than I was as a factory manager. I relied on staffs of analysts to tell me what people wanted; you don't have those resources. I rarely met my customers; you see and touch yours daily. I wouldn't have known how to respond to end-user complaints; your job is to do precisely that.

Some would say your best-selling service is transportation. I'd argue it's compassion, and you're in charge of its quality and distribution.

One would think exceptional service would be emphasized throughout face-to-face industries like ours. I haven't found that to be the case. I bet you have just as many stories as I do about arrogant, self-indulgent EMTs, paramedics, doctors, and nurses, so I'll add one about a medical office whose staff must have been absent the day they covered patient-provider synergy in administrator school:

When my health insurer stopped paying for lab work done outside my home state, I went to my family physician's practice—a large, suburban facility—to ask that all specimens donated by me be sent to any of the local laboratories on my plan's list. I already knew my doctor used two of those labs, so I wasn't expecting trouble.

I hadn't even finished my request when I noticed the receptionist cracking her knuckles. I thought, *this is bad.* I also thought, *wow, that's the first time I've seen a woman crack her knuckles.*

When my alleged service provider told me how little she could do for me, I asked for someone with more responsibility and, if possible, more tact. I found the former but not the latter; the second employee's manner was equally unsympathetic.

I don't know if rudeness is a prerequisite for workers at that office, but I'm pretty sure the answers I got had more to do with two burned-out bureaucrats who tried to trivialize me rather than help me. In my tormentors' world, I wasn't entitled to their deference because I hadn't "paid my dues"—i.e., I hadn't experienced *their* frustrations in *their* workplace.

Have I ever treated patients that way? Yes, perhaps a dozen in 20 years. Then there are those whose needs I could have met more effectively by setting aside protocols and concentrating on what those folks were trying to tell me. I struggle with such subtle, subjective elements of care every day. I'm constantly reminding myself I'm there to serve people, not the reverse. Along the way, I've tried to embrace these critical aspects of customer relations:

When to serve. Right away, according to careerealism.com, which estimates we have less than 30 seconds to impress each other. *Psychology Today* credits eye contact, a pleasant mood, reciprocal gestures, and an unforced smile as key elements of favorable first encounters.

How to serve. When possible, let our patients tell us. High-frequency listening is a skill some of us lack but all of us can learn.

Why serve? Because medicine isn't just an intellectual exercise. It's easy to become preoccupied with the scripted science of medical emergencies, but the S in EMS reminds us that service is what we're selling.

The exceptional among us have already embraced those principles. For them, being nice to people is a natural act. They purposefully relate to their patients because they've seen how bedside anonymity hinders customized care. Our finest already know that prompt, compassionate, unflappable service with so much at stake distinguishes even the least experienced EMS provider from those who work at something less.

LIFE AFTER EMS

2018

I remember the moment I knew I was done with EMS.

Four months after my last back injury, I was treating a middle-aged male in rapid a-fib. He was symptomatic enough to warrant rate control, if not cardioversion. Kneeling on the floor to start an IV—something I'd done hundreds of times—was awkward and painful because my left leg wasn't working right. Even worse was trying to stand up after the stick. I probably looked like I needed an ambulance as much as my patient, but all I wanted at that instant was to walk away from EMS with some dignity. I was 60.

That was five years ago. I've spent the last four of them missing field work so much, I tease myself about absurd circumstances that would allow me to go back—like finding a 9-1-1 job that exempted me from bending, lifting, and carrying. Imagine how popular I'd be with my partners.

An Atypical Path

Despite my abbreviated career as a caregiver, I feel pretty lucky compared to some of my coworkers. At least EMS wasn't the only thing I ever wanted to do. I didn't chase fire engines as a kid and wasn't an *Emergency!* junkie in the '70s, mostly because I wanted to make more money than the Johnny Gages of the world. I went to engineering school and worked in the cosmetics/pharmaceuticals industry, where the pay was fine, but the politics were brutal.

I was good at my jobs—a new one every few years—but too much of a maverick to curry favor with the right people. I broke rules and was outspoken about doing so. I moved up the corporate ladder, but not as quickly as some of my better-behaved colleagues. After 14 years of working for others, I started consulting full time to see if being my own boss would help me find the contentment of the gainfully employed I'd been seeking since college. It didn't.

In 1993, I shifted my focus to EMS, became a paramedic in 1995, and gained the job satisfaction that had been so elusive. What I didn't have was an exit strategy—a plan for leaving EMS either by choice or chance. Now that I'm working through that exercise, maybe I can help you prepare for the same.

Catecholamine Crisis

The first thing I noticed about being away from EMS was weight gain. For 20 years, I'd carried only 140-145 pounds on my skinny 5'9" frame, but by 2015—two years after leaving—I was close to 180. At first, I thought it was because I was getting less exercise—a factor, no doubt, but not the main reason for needing a bigger belt.

As much as I'd enjoyed working clinically, I rarely felt as calm as my partners seemed. While they'd rant about, say, the symbiotic relationship between burgers and beer, I'd ponder the call we'd just had. Those weren't unpleasant thoughts; for me, mentally cataloging the good and bad was a natural act. Even on days off, I'd play what-if with high-stakes scenarios and try to simulate the buzz that accompanied difficult cases.

Feeling excited about EMS kept me motivated and engaged, but also on edge. I'm pretty sure those free-flowing catecholamines were most responsible for my loose pants all those years. I mention that not as a wardrobe issue, but as a warning that one of the biggest consequences of leaving the field can be metabolic.

What can you do about that? Lots more than I did. Exercise and diet should be no-brainers, but I had trouble with both. It's hard to suddenly start eating healthy after years of deep-fried, super-sized sustenance. Eventually, I limited myself to one full meal a day and a light snack. As for staying active, the sports I used to enjoy most—hockey, racquetball, and bowling—were out because of my back. Even walking more than a few hundred feet at a time became a problem. Exercise is still a work in progress, although my weight just passed 175 on the way down, thanks to portion control at mealtime and some chores around the house.

The mental adjustment has been much more challenging for me, as I am now a paramedic in name only.

Chasing an Image

I was once asked at a 1980s job interview, "Who is Mike Rubin?" Even allowing for the interviewer's wacky technique, it was a great question. I answered with something like, "A manager, an engineer."

"No, no," my prospective employer said, "not *what* are you. *Who* are you?"

I find it hard to separate the two. I still see myself as a paramedic although I haven't had a clinical job in five years. It helps to live in Tennessee, where I can be a medic as long as I meet continuing-education requirements, pay application fees, and don't commit felonies.

I tell myself I'm keeping my license because it gives me more credibility as a writer. Perhaps, but the real reason is that it makes me feel better to wake up each morning with a hard-earned title—one I feel differentiates me from the minions of white-collar culture. If I gave up that distinction, I'd just be some old guy with creepy stories.

I do know I'm not a *real* paramedic. They have patients. My last was in 2013. Comparing myself to those of you still in the field makes me feel phony, yet every two years I go to class, send money to the state, and promise myself that's the last time.

I'll tell you when my final recert will be: when I gratefully settle for not having maimed or killed anyone during two decades in EMS and take pride in just being a husband, father, and grandfather. That's a work in progress, too.

Filling in the Blanks

Most of us don't move seamlessly from EMS to something else. There's often a period when cash flow is interrupted, or at least slowed. Getting past that requires a hands-on approach to money management including, for many, a much better understanding of Social Security and Medicare. I say that because I was surprised to learn how much I didn't know about those programs.

Uncle Sam gives us options and rights. Confuse those two and you could end up outliving your means. Details about that and other financial complexities are beyond the scope of this article, but well within the reach of these books:

- *Get What's Yours* by Laurence Kotlikoff, Philip Moeller, and Paul Solman. This is *the* definitive user guide for Social Security. Despite the tedious subject matter, it's folksy and even amusing, with lots of real-world examples.
- *Get What's Yours for Medicare* by Philip Moeller. Similar in style to the above, but focusing on Medicare.
- *Retirement Planning Made Easy* by Diane Marra. Written by an ex-paramedic who succeeded at life after EMS as a financial consultant.

Leveraging EMS

You're probably wondering, *So Mike, what am I supposed to do while I work toward all those endpoints you've never reached?* Maybe think about what you're good at after so many years in the field, and how you can leverage that talent.

This is where EMS providers are at a disadvantage compared to firefighters and LEOs. The world has become a target-rich environment for hazmat and security consultants. EMS specialists? Not so much. The best-paying gig for retired paramedics is probably expert-witness work, but few of us have the connections to make that happen.

What most ex-paramedics do have is command presence, street smarts, and the ability to handle pressure. All those qualities have value elsewhere in industry. It's up to you to accentuate your "very particular set of skills" when exploring post-EMS opportunities.

What did you like best about EMS? For me, it was problem solving and working largely unsupervised. I found going back to consulting and focusing on writing satisfied some of those cravings. I'm not having as much fun as I did answering calls, and I'm still looking for that "unconscious, not breathing" buzz, but at least I'm paying bills and not burdening my family with a woe-is-me attitude . . . well, hardly ever.

If you're ambitious enough to seek another occupation that has at least some of the qualities you loved about EMS, do research, take courses, read books. It helps to be young with money, but I wouldn't bet against anyone who thrived in the patient-care business.

I'll be right behind you.

SPIRITUALITY IN EMS

2012

The dawn was like no other, distinguished not by a rescue gone right, but by the view from the end of a steel cable a hundred feet above Tennessee's Roaring River. Paramedic Chris Masiongale marveled at smoldering sunlight piercing summer mist as he and Sean Buckley, a 23-year-old medic with the 50th Medical Company of the 8th Battalion, 101st Airborne, were hoisted toward the UH-60 Blackhawk, a helicopter whose military exploits overshadow its peacetime role as a medevac platform.

It had been a long night for Chris and his fellow responders. The search for hikers Ralph Hayes and his son, Joel, near the intersection of Jackson, Putnam, and Overton counties in north-central Tennessee started six hours earlier. Both men had been found on the riverbank suffering from tib/fib fractures and hypothermia. Rough terrain complicated conventional transport, so Chris's supervisor called the MAST (Military Assistance, Safety, Traffic) unit at Fort Campbell on the Kentucky border for assistance. After airlifting the injured to a local hospital, the soldiers had returned to pick up Masiongale and Leon Harris, another rescuer.

As the Blackhawk hovered above, Buckley was lowered to the ground by a starboard-side winch. The Army medic had advised Masiongale and Harris he could take only one of them at a time. The 29-year-old Masiongale, who'd never been in a helicopter, reluctantly agreed to go first.

Buckley and Masiongale sat facing each other on the penetrator, a three-legged lifting device resembling a blunt, inverted grappling hook. Sean's legs straddled Chris's torso in a minimalist arrangement requiring

*a mutual embrace for support. Superficial shoulder straps added psycho-
logical, more than functional, protection.*

*The 10-by-15-foot rock that had been their launch pad receded
beneath the medics' boots as the shriek of two General Electric
1,890-horsepower turboshafts overwhelmed the whine of the winch. At
the treetops seconds later, Chris lauded the panorama afforded by the
gentle rotation of the penetrator. "What a beautiful view," he said. Sean
didn't respond. To Chris, he seemed preoccupied.*

What is spirituality? My dictionary defines it as "religious devotion
or piety; the rights, jurisdiction, tithes, etc. belonging to the church or
to an ecclesiastic." Most of the EMS providers I interviewed for this
article disagreed spirituality is necessarily linked to religion or houses
of worship. "The side of personality that's all good," "the ability to
connect to yourself and loved ones," "the way you frame your world,"
and "how you live your life" are concepts of spirituality asserted by
prehospital practitioners during eight hours of discussion. However,
secular views weren't the only sentiments expressed. "Showing your
faith," "going to church," and "belief in God" are other definitions of
spirituality voiced by our colleagues. It seems there is no more of an
EMS consensus on spirituality than on ambulance configuration.

Why, then, tackle a topic as subjective as spirituality? There are no
practical exams to evaluate spiritual skills. The word isn't even mentioned in any of my textbooks. According to my state's prehospital
protocols, spirituality is less of a concern than application of MAST
pants, packaging of avulsed teeth, and transportation of dead snakes.
Is spirituality a subject best relinquished to clerics?

I might have settled for that outcome had I not read a story by com-
mentator Robert Krulwich about Richard Feynman, an American
physicist who helped develop the atom bomb. Feynman was at the
bedside of his terminally ill wife when she died of Hodgkin's disease.
According to Krulwich, Feynman noticed that the clock on the wall
of his wife's hospital room had stopped at 9:21 PM, the precise time
of her death. The physicist saw no significance in that; the clock had
been broken and fixed before. He reasoned someone had jostled the
fragile timepiece, causing it to malfunction again.

Krulwich suggests many of us would see a link between the
stopped clock and the death of Feynman's wife. "I know how the

story would feel to me," he says. "It would be as though the universe had somehow noticed what had happened; that some invisible hand slipped into my world and pointed, as if to say, 'We know. This is part of the plan.'"

As I continued my interviews, I heard repeated references to such a plan. Called "God's will" by some and "a master plan" by others, the belief "everything happens for a reason" was nearly unanimous. I concluded, if so many EMS providers agree on that aspect of spirituality, most of the people we care for probably would, too. Spirituality, then, might be more than just a personal conviction; it could be a shared experience that connects caregivers to patients. I don't know of any medicine that causes that. I think that's reason enough to explore spirituality in EMS.

One more thing: As I was editing the above paragraph, my watch broke. I'm not kidding. The band around my wrist separated spontaneously from the timepiece. No, it hadn't been broken and fixed before. No, it wasn't jostled.

"Something's wrong," Buckley screamed at Masiongale over the roar of the Blackhawk's rotor.

"What?" Chris yelled back. He could only lip-read what his fellow medic said.

"Something's wrong!" Sean shouted again.

Forty feet below the chopper's skids, the counterclockwise rotation of the rescuers about the cable had become more pronounced. Chris didn't know their coiled lifeline was fraying after repeated contact with the helicopter's titanium hull. Sean realized they were in trouble and was trying to signal Chris over the cacophony of the engines.

Masiongale looked up at the Blackhawk's open hatch, saw the winch operator struggling to corral the cable, then grasped reflexively at one of the skids, which seemed no more than an arm's length above. The crewman at the winch reached down toward Chris. Both knew the gesture was futile.

Spirituality and the practice of medicine are linked in Judeo-Christian literature. According to medical historian Henry Sigerist,

Christianity began as a "religion of healing." Christians were urged to tend to the sick and view the suffering of others as a greater concern than their own misfortunes.

Judaism proclaimed our bodies are God's property, loaned to us. Protecting that property takes priority over every commandment except those prohibiting incest, idolatry, and murder. The Talmud, Judaism's sacred compilation of customs and laws, forbids Jews to live in cities that have no physicians.

Unfortunately, pre-medieval populations had little to offer each other in times of illness. Purveyors of oils, charms, and chants competed with the earliest physicians for recognition as healers. Jews, Christians, and pagans often turned to "magical" cures when primitive science failed to relieve disability and disease. Herbs, amulets, and spells were no less effective than rudimentary medicine, which boasted therapeutics such as urine-spiked cocktails and bloodletting.

By the Middle Ages, the Catholic Church was becoming frustrated with practitioners of folk medicine who failed to credit God as the ultimate healer. Theologians, many of whom were serving as de facto physicians, urged medical professionals to evaluate patients' spirituality before delivering care. Medieval patient interviews were as much about determining compliance with Church doctrines as assessing chief complaints.

The Protestant Reformation sparked a shift in how the sciences, including medicine, were viewed. Martin Luther, a leader of the Reformation, favored inductive reasoning based on experience over adherence to written rules. Luther, who suffered from numerous maladies throughout his adult life, urged doctors to learn their craft through fieldwork, yet reminded them faith and prayer were essential elements of their practice. "I have nothing but praise for the physicians who adhere closely to their principles," he said, "but they shouldn't take it amiss if I don't always agree with them . . ."

John Calvin, another 16th-century Protestant leader, acclaimed God as the "great physician" while defending doctors against those who saw medicine as the enterprise of evil spirits. "Anyone with an ounce of brains knows (physicians) are gifts of God," he wrote.

Calvin joined Luther in urging establishment of government-funded hospitals. The symbiosis of medicine and theology is further corroborated by the dual cleric-physician pedigrees of new-world

Protestant reformers John Clarke (Baptist), Francis Makemie (Presbyterian), Henry Melchior Muhlenberg (Lutheran), and Samuel Seabury (Episcopal).

> *Masiongale and Buckley were 175 feet above the Roaring River when the cable hoisting them into the helicopter snapped just above their heads. Masiongale heard a loud* crack! *like a shotgun blast, accompanied by the sudden mushrooming of steel strands. "I was scared to death," Chris recalls. "Then it got real quiet."*
>
> *According to Masiongale, the old saying about seeing your life flash before you is true. "It was like I took a deep breath and everything was calm. I was thinking about my childhood, my family, my kids, positive influences in my life, and a disagreement I'd just had with my partner, Beck. I know that sounds like a lot, but it all went through my mind on the way down. For me, it was a very long fall.*
>
> *"I figured we'd hit those same rocks we'd just lifted off of. I never expected to live through it."*

Why do bad things happen to good people?

That question is a test of faith for some caregivers and a point of contention for others.

"In May of 1981, we had a house fire in Cherry Hill [New Jersey]," recalls John Fleischmann, paramedic and Lutheran minister. "Four children died. I still have dreams about that.

"What do you say to people who lose all their kids in the blink of an eye? We can't answer why. From my point of view, it just makes you want to trust God more. We can't see the whole picture; we only see a little sliver every day.

"Just because you have faith doesn't mean you're immune from suffering. Everyone suffers—some more than others."

EMT Karen Lambert and her paramedic husband, Rob, remember a horrific motor vehicle accident involving a mother and three teenagers.

"When I got there, [the first responders] were doing CPR on the mother," Rob recalls. "All three kids were unresponsive, still in the car. I told [the responders] to stop working on the mother so we could try to save the others.

"The daughter died before we could get her out of the car. The son and his friend were in bad shape. I didn't expect either of them to make it.

"A couple of years later, we were called to the home of a wheelchair-bound patient with sepsis. It turned out to be the son. According to his father, the boy hadn't been able to do much since the accident. I felt terrible, thinking we'd made a mistake trying to save his life, but his father thanked us and said, after losing the rest of his family, his son is all that keeps him going. That made me feel better."

Dealing with misfortune is "a major concept in Judaism" according to Rachel "Ruchie" Freier, who founded *Ezras Nashim* (Hebrew for "assisting women"), a Brooklyn-based EMS corps composed entirely of Hasidic women. "God has a master plan. We're not always privy to it. It's like life is a color picture we're seeing in black and white. That doesn't diminish my belief in God. I know I'm here for a purpose and I'm going to do the best I can."

Some dispute any presumption of purpose to hardship. Consider this anonymous comment: "Shortly after becoming a paramedic, I had a bad call where a child died because of neglect. I asked several religious people and even the pastor at my church why God would allow such a thing to happen. He said God works in mysterious ways and has a plan for each of us. He also said bad things happen to good people for no reason. I know that. I didn't need him to tell me that."

My wife, Helen, who just retired after a long career in the essential services, has a different take on the topic: "Bad things happen to all people—not just good people. Good things also happen to good and bad people. It's up to us to make the best of all situations."

Less than four seconds after their cable broke, Buckley and Masiongale landed between jagged rocks in a 40-square-foot pool of water not more than two feet deep. They had been falling at over 70 miles an hour. "I can't tell you what it was like to hit because I don't remember," Chris says. "I think God spared me that experience. Whenever I woke up, I was underwater."

Leon Harris, the rescuer left behind who would have been evacuated after Chris, was facing away from the helicopter when the line snapped. Harris felt water on his back, turned around and realized Sean and Chris had made that splash. He jumped in the river and grabbed a medic in each hand, struggling to hold their heads above water. The swift current tugged at Buckley and Masiongale. Harris knew he'd soon have to decide which one to let go.

Spirituality in EMS is as much about patients as providers, according to colleagues.

"Lots of times, people forget the spiritual part of first aid is just as important as dressing a wound or starting an IV," Fleischmann says. "I think everyone has the capability to put patients at ease. Some are better at it than others, but it's something we can all work on.

"Just take the risk and start a conversation with a patient. You can be spiritual without getting into technicalities about faith."

Kentucky paramedic Kevin Hurley thinks honesty is an important part of spirituality. "I had this young girl who got run over. She tried to commit suicide by lying in the middle of the road. When we got there, she was all busted up.

"'Am I going to make it?' she asked. I said no, I don't think so, but it's not up to me.

"'What should I do? I think I made a mistake.' I told her to make her peace with God. He'll decide the next step.

"She prayed out loud and calmed down. Then she died in the OR."

Fleischmann agrees it's not our job to judge patients. "We'd get calls almost every night for a guy supposedly having a seizure. He'd be talking when our crews got there, so everyone assumed he was faking. Turns out he was having a dystonic reaction to his medication. Nobody realized that because they were so busy judging him."

We shouldn't underestimate the therapeutic value of kindness, according to this anonymous account:

"My mother had a major heart attack in 1998. During the trip to the hospital, her heart stopped twice. The EMT not only resuscitated her, but kept talking to her, reassuring her while she was unconscious. She heard it all. When she recovered, she wrote him a letter to thank him for all the encouragement.

"Several years later, after Mom had moved a couple hundred miles away, she had another heart attack. Who showed up? That same EMT! He had moved, too.

"Mom passed away last week. There were two eulogies—one from my brother and one from Mom's 'favorite EMT.'"

Leon Harris was spared the toughest decision of his life by eight members of the Overton County Rescue Squad who had not gotten an earlier message to return to headquarters. They helped Harris pull the semiconscious medics onto the riverbank and did what they could to stabilize grave injuries: Buckley had bilateral hip, femur, and tib/fib fractures. Masiongale's back was broken in three places, all of the ribs on his right side were shattered, and every bone in his face was fractured. Pain isn't what he remembers, though.

"I was angry," the Byrdstown, Tennessee native says. "Angry at being hurt, angry at being alive. I'd already accepted the fact I was going to die. I thought, 'This doesn't make any sense.'"

Then Masiongale heard a voice next to his right ear.

"Chris, it's okay." The pitch was male, the tone clear and reassuring. "Everything's going to be alright, but you have to decide whether you're going to live or die. There's no shame in either."

Masiongale didn't want to have to choose. "I'd already decided on the way down I wasn't going to live. I'd made peace with that. Now I was in every kind of shock you can think of and just wanted to let go. But that voice called me back. I still don't know where it came from.

"I started bargaining with myself: 'Well, let's not make the decision yet, because there are some people I need to talk to.'"

According to the Lamberts, spirituality in EMS extends to personal lives. "Rob and I have been through a lot in our marriage," Karen says. "EMS takes time away from us. Sometimes it tests our relationship. But in the long run, I think it makes us stronger."

Larry Zacarese, a New York paramedic and third-generation police officer, seconds the importance of family support.

"I was a new medic when one of my partners committed suicide. One day she switched tours to get supplies for a lidocaine/potassium drip. The next day she killed herself with it. It was a shock. It ran against everything we're supposed to do.

"I'm lucky my wife is in the field. You need to have outlets. You need to be able to talk about [bad calls]."

Fleischmann sees balance as a key to spirituality. "It's important to have a life outside of EMS, to be able to turn off that built-in duty to act we all feel.

"To be a good EMS provider, you have to be a whole person."

Wendy Holt, a Tennessee EMT-IV, says she's not the same person she was before EMS. "I had nothing. I never thought I'd be able to provide for my family. EMS made me stronger by making my faith stronger. If you have faith, you have everything."

Jim Morgan, Masiongale's usual partner, had been off duty but close by when the medics fell. He rushed to the scene and found a path through the brush for the responding vehicles. Chris was carried to a waiting ambulance, then had a moment alone with Beck, the medic he'd argued with earlier. "It was very quiet in back—just the two of us. I grabbed hold of her hand and said, 'I have to tell you, I'm sorry. I want things to be okay between us.' I could tell it upset her, but she stayed professional and did her job.

"I don't remember any pain on the way to the hospital."

Fifteen minutes later, Chris was in Trauma Room 1 at Livingston Hospital surrounded by ED staff. "They were having trouble starting IVs. I'd lost a lot of blood," Masiongale recalls.

Chris's wife, Malissa, was by his right side. "I still didn't think I'd survive. I said my good-byes. Then they brought in my little girl (two-year-old Kaylee). She looked down at me and started crying. I reached up and grabbed her hand. That's when I decided I was going to live. I told her I'd be okay.

"Then I started hurting."

Chris Masiongale was flown to Erlanger Medical Center in Chattanooga, where he received eight units of whole blood, four units of platelets, and four of plasma. Doctors expected him to be hospitalized for several weeks at least, but he was discharged in six days. He attributes his rapid recovery to prayer and "wanting to get back to Kaylee."

"There's no medical reason a man who's lost every bit of blood in his body should still be alive," he says. "I don't know why. I don't think I'm supposed to know why. I'm just thankful for the chance to enjoy the world around me—my family, the sky, opening presents Christmas morning. I've learned to appreciate the little things. I try to share that feeling with my patients."

Masiongale's tale highlights the message of colleagues, theologians, and historians: Caring for others is the essence of spirituality. EMS providers can demonstrate that spirit by embracing our roles as caregivers, strengthening ourselves through faith, and showing compassion to anyone having a bad day. These are principles, not protocols; they aren't stowed like boots or bags after shifts. Spirituality in EMS is an extension of spirituality in life.

Consider this incident:

An elderly female stumbles and falls in front of a strip mall. There are many witnesses, but only one responds—a retired EMS worker, who finds no major injuries. The patient refuses an ambulance; her chief complaint is broken eyeglasses. "How am I going to get home?" she wails. "I can't drive without my glasses." None of the woman's family is available, so the ex-EMT offers to drive her to a nearby optometrist. The patient gratefully accepts. Forty minutes later, her eyeglasses are fixed and she's back in her car, bruised but mobile.

The good Samaritan in that story is Helen. I think her self-imposed duty to act is as spiritually vivid as any services we can hope to provide on the job. When we put EMS aside at the end of a day or a career, our bias to care offers spiritual continuity. Procedures and policies become less important than remembering what it feels like to be a rescuer.

IN CASE YOU'RE INTERESTED . . .

EARLY PATIENT ASSESSMENT

2018

My first practical exercise as a soon-to-be-EMT began when my instructor said something like, "You respond to a 25-year-old female complaining of abdominal pain. Take it from there." That was my cue to declare "The scene is safe," or maybe "I'm wearing PPE"—two fewer reasons to fail that station automatically (as opposed to failing it with maximum effort).

I figured scene safety and personal protective equipment were most important because they were right at the top of New York's patient-assessment skill sheets for both medical and trauma scenarios. What I didn't yet know—how could I?—is that prompt, accurate assessment requires imagination and flexibility much more than memorization of sequential to-do lists.

It's hard to practice assessment scenarios without making EMS seem more scientific than it is. Look at the National Registry's advanced-level psychomotor exam, for example: The skill sheet for assessment of medical patients includes 39 competencies, 37 of which are perfunctory steps characterized by straightforward verbs such as *determines, verbalizes, questions,* and *repeats.* Only two interventions— *Considers stabilization of spine* and *Evaluates response to treatments*— imply open-ended judgment.

Judgment is precisely what drives assessment—at least it should. Real cases almost never follow the predictable patterns of classroom exercises. Instead, the outcome of each action indicates the next one. The clearest example of that is the patient interview.

What's Going On?

Interviewing has been a big part of my job for almost 50 years, as a journalist and EMS provider. Way back in the beginning, the best advice I got about interviewing was to pursue whatever made me curious—not as a reporter or a paramedic, but as a person.

Consider an encounter with someone who's obviously sick or injured. Even without medical training, you'd wonder what was going on. Ask a question as if you were assessing a family member instead of a patient.

"What's going on?" is even consistent with the scientific method, not that science is as useful during an interview as high-frequency listening—paying attention to answers and body language while forming appropriate follow-up questions. That's hard to do if you get distracted by mnemonics or algorithms. For example, if the 25-year-old in my opening paragraph told me her belly hurt, the next thing I'd want to know is where. That's pretty important for abdominal complaints, but you won't find a *W* for *where* or any close equivalent in OPQRST or SAMPLE.

My priority during assessment is to determine how emergent the presenting problem is and whether treatment or transport should come first. The best field practitioners I know make those decisions in 30-60 seconds. To do so requires a healthy regard for what we *can't* do in an ambulance.

Be conservative. We're not doctors and very few of us have pre-hospital access to imaging. Initiating transport to definitive-care facilities is usually the right call, except when outcomes are so time dependent (e.g., cardiac arrests) that delaying treatment even a few minutes can be fatal.

Low-Tech Multitasking

The most important assessment tools are our brains and senses. We're blessed to be able to use them in parallel; to palpate a pulse, for example, while interviewing a patient.

Notice I said palpate. You don't need wires, clamps, or batteries for that. Pulse oximeters and cardiac monitors show pulse rate but not pulse character—fast or slow, weak or strong, regular or irregular, regularly irregular or irregularly irregular. Each is a noteworthy clue during assessment.

When I was answering calls, I'd gently borrow the wrist of my patient almost as soon as I greeted its owner. While feeling the pulse, I'd also observe the character of

- respirations: fast or slow, noisy or quiet, labored or unlabored?
- pupils: big or small, equal or unequal, aligned or not?
- skin: trauma, color, and moisture.

None of that requires digital displays. All of it can be done while conversing with responsive patients.

What basic assessment information haven't we mentioned? Blood pressure, O_2 saturation, and lung sounds. All involve equipment—not a problem if you have it, but still subordinate to what you see, hear, and feel. For the most excellent among us, measurable anomalies during assessment merely support initial impressions.

Horses versus Zebras

I bet every industry has sayings as tiresome as, *When you hear hoofbeats, think horses, not zebras.* Enough, already—we get it: The most likely diagnoses are usually the correct ones.

And yet . . .

What if your patient's illness has more than one cause? Is there anything about your assessment that doesn't fit your conclusions? Might you be hearing a zebra instead of a horse?

In his book, *How Doctors Think,* Jerome Groopman, MD, suggests physicians consider the above questions to discourage hasty pattern-matching or confirmation bias. If doctors make those kinds of mistakes, EMS providers can too—especially when an assessment leads to ambiguous findings.

A subtle but important element of diagnosing is to keep an open mind about less-likely possibilities. A good example is the trauma victim who turns out to be hypoglycemic. I've seen about a dozen cases of AMS blamed on a mechanism of injury, when low blood sugar was the cause. When forming conclusions during assessment, don't hesitate to consider what else it could be.

Art versus Science

The argument that patient assessment should be driven more by experience and flexibility than skill sheets and circuitry isn't controversial or new. We're merely suggesting there are no machines capable of evaluating illness and injury as insightfully as people. That's not a knock on technology—just a reminder that digital interpretations of an analog world are necessarily limited. How we sense and surmise what's ailing our patients is an art form that can be supported by science, but not replaced by it.

THE
LOW-MAINTENANCE
EMPLOYEE

2018

For those of you active in the job market, I have some surprising news about prospective employers: They're not too worried about your skills, experience, appearance, or ability to get along with others. They don't care if you go to church or volunteer at the local rescue squad. Their main concern—pretty much the only one they've had since interviewing you—is "What can you do for me?"

That might sound selfish and short-sighted, but it hints at the implicit contract between fair bosses and their subordinates: you take care of me and I'll take care of you. Your part—to make life as easy as possible for the people who pay you—means embracing the quiet confidence and relative anonymity of low-maintenance employees.

When Grades Aren't as Simple as ABC

Getting hired in EMS is a legitimate reason to celebrate. For many, it's an opportunity to turn a passion into a career. That's about as good as it gets when you're working for someone else. That "dream job" can be a big adjustment, though—especially for new EMTs with little paid experience. Suddenly, EMS isn't primarily a social or recreational activity; it's a responsibility involving long hours and obligatory attendance.

Even more of a challenge for those fresh out of school is the difference between academia's unambiguous report cards and the subtler performance measures of the business community. Gone are the days of getting credit merely for showing up. As for those test-taking skills that earned you As and Bs instead of Cs and Ds, they'll still come in handy when you recertify, but won't count for much else.

Welcome to Working for a Living, where standing out doesn't necessarily make you outstanding. Your stock as a corporate asset will rise if you are inconspicuously competent and fall if you inconvenience others. To succeed, you don't even have to be a great clinician, although that helps. Being accommodating—not a natural act for some—is important whether your company's organization chart is highly structured or hardly defined.

Low-Maintenance and Low-Profile

We're talking about being accommodating, not servile. Your goal is to establish mutually beneficial relationships with your bosses: job security in exchange for your cooperation. During downtime, when it's easiest for an employer to evaluate you in person, start building a rapport by following these steps:

- **Say what you'll do, then do what you said.** This is good advice for any endeavor. Routinely committing to a course of action and seeing it through automatically makes you more reliable than most human beings.
- **Become "assistant risk manager."** Mostly, that means telling your employer about problems before they get any bigger. The stakes are higher in business than in the academic world, where students only have to look out for themselves.
- **Don't screw up, but if you do, tell your boss.** When you make a mistake, don't wait for your supervisor to find out from someone else. Admitting an error adds to your credibility and shows you are capable of self-critique—probably more important than whatever you messed up.
- **Come to management with solutions, not just problems.** We're talking about issues less challenging than, say, nuclear proliferation. Take drug bags: Meds expire, vials break, and stuff gets lost in compartments you didn't even know existed. Instead of complaining, suggest a better layout.

- **Be early, stay late.** Do that, and you'll impress not only your employers, but your peers. If you rounded up all my ex-partners and asked them what they liked best about me (besides my Germanic charm), I bet they'd say it was arriving 10–15 minutes early for almost every shift.
- **Be reasonable.** When you and your supervisor disagree, think long-term and show willingness to compromise. You'll get no points just for winning an argument.
- **Become the one your boss depends on.** If you're new to EMS, most of your colleagues will know more than you about the job, but you're going to be more flexible and less cynical than them—in the beginning, at least. During that first year of eagerness, when channeling your inner Johnny Gage is as natural as buckling your buff belt, be that guy or gal who volunteers for extra shifts, tedious errands, and whatever else no one wants to do. I promise you, your employer will value you ahead of more experienced but less cooperative coworkers.

Good clinicians are appreciated; trustworthy, low-maintenance employees are treasured. Come to work with a purpose, be available and dependable, let your actions speak louder than words, and your boss may even ask, "What can *I* do for *you*?"

ON THE MONEY

2017

I was catching up with online comments from the EMS community when I spotted this post:

> I've looked at job listings and I see most EMT-B jobs (in suburban Chicago) state either $12/hr or $25K a year with medical/dental benefits. Is anyone else able to fully cover their living expenses from a single source of income in that range?

What concerned me about that question even more than its affirmation of subsistence-level wages in EMS was the author's apparent uncertainty about his own solvency, and the extent to which he thought others could help. That's like polling coworkers to see which uniform fits best. Wait, I've seen that, too.

Money management is a domestic skill like carpentry or plumbing—natural acts for some, nightmares for others. Take me, for example; I'm fine with finances mostly because I was the kid who always saved more than he spent. If I got a few bucks for my birthday, it went into the bank because I liked to watch the numbers in that passbook grow. Ask me to fix a leaky faucet, though, and we're going to need a bigger boat.

I think most EMTs and paramedics would rather dig a well through bedrock than spend that time balancing their books. I'm not sure why; maybe money seems confusing because we tend to have so little of it. Deconstructing life paycheck by paycheck doesn't leave many decisions about saving. However, needing almost every dime for urgencies makes it even more important to understand at least a few bookkeeping basics:

Budgeting

Every adult should estimate their annual income versus expenses at least once a year. It's called budgeting—something that used to be second nature for anyone not named Rockefeller.

The consequences of ignoring one's own bottom line can be severe —overdrawn accounts, massive credit-card debt, even bankruptcy. For many in EMS, though, budgeting is harder than high-stakes patient care. It doesn't have to be.

Start by estimating expenses monthly or even annually. Pick general categories, such as clothing, insurance, and food. Drilling down to meat, fish, and eggs is reserved for psychotic engineer/paramedic/columnists from Boston.

Round to the nearest $100. Be conservative; better to overstate expenses than to understate them. If you're comfortable using a spreadsheet like Excel, fine; otherwise, pencil, paper, and a calculator will work just as well.

When you're finished with that part, you'll have a list of categories something like this: cars, clothing, dental, dues, electricity, entertainment, food, furnishings, gasoline, gifts, grooming, hobbies, housewares, insurance, maintenance, medical, postage, publications, telephone, travel, water, and other, with dollar figures next to them. Add those up. That's your nut. Covering it depends on after-tax income, but taxes aren't the only deductions that lighten your paycheck. Find a pay stub from each of your current jobs, then read on.

Deductions

The difference between earnings and take-home pay can be a source of confusion, not to mention irritation. Allow yourself two minutes for an Orwellian rant against big brother, then review your deductions dispassionately. Although wages withheld count as income, you might not be taking home enough to pay bills.

The most common payroll mistake I've seen working people make is withholding too much for taxes. The idea of a big, annual tax refund seems to be more appealing than using those funds during the year. Can you say, "strategic blunder"? I knew you could.

Those tax-refund "windfalls" mean you've made an interest-free loan to the federal government—and to your state and city, in some cases. Even the low interest rates you'd get for banking those sums is better than nothing, which is what you'll earn from tax collectors who use your money.

If you deduct too little, you'll face even bigger problems in the form of interest and penalties. The trick is to adjust withholding so that year-end tax due is as close to zero as possible. And don't listen to coworkers who complain about the government taking almost all of their overtime pay. Those wages aren't treated any differently by the IRS than the first dollar you earn each year.

Taxes aren't the only obligations coming out of paychecks. Most employees have to share the cost of medical insurance. Some pay for dental or disability, too. Deductions for savings plans such as 401Ks are also common. In general, it makes sense to contribute as much as you can to those tax-advantaged investments while leaving enough to cover your bills. What you don't want to do is make up the difference with credit card debt. As of this writing, the average interest rate on unpaid balances is over 15%. It would be hard to come up with a worse long-term investment strategy than borrowing heavily with plastic. I would be happy to lend you money at half that rate and use your interest to finance an oceanfront bungalow in Tahiti, assuming I can watch hockey in Tahiti.

Dollars and Sense

My friend Tom Bouthillet is an EKG expert. We're talking physician-level, even though Tom's a paramedic. Most medics don't have anywhere near Tom's mastery of EKGs, but that doesn't mean we don't use our more modest 12-lead skills to help care for patients.

Managing money is similar: You don't have to be an expert to make good decisions. Learn the basics, appreciate what you don't know, and review income versus expenses at least a few times a year. You'll have more control and fewer surprises.

Author's Note

Money management goals change as we age—at least they should. So do tactics. When you're young, you have a better chance of riding out stock-market downturns and erasing paper losses during prosperous times to come.

Transitioning from wealth-building to preservation of assets is something many of us face as we age. The key is managing risk—a skill not at all foreign to EMS providers.

KEEPING THE SCENE SERENE

2016

In 1995, not quite three months into my paramedic career, my partner Donna and I responded to a diabetic emergency. The patient, a brawny, combative, insulin-dependent male, was brandishing a length of pipe.

I knew from the man's daughter that her dad had probably over-medicated himself. He'd done so before with the same outcome. The situation called for a strategic retreat until the police could be summoned, but I was still basking in the confidence of my new paramedic-ness, and was intrigued at the possibility of convincing our patient to put down his hunk of hardware so I could give him glucose. I moved closer, not all that mindful of danger.

Fortunately, Donna had called for help as soon as we got there. Arriving even before the cops was Andy, one of our most experienced EMTs, who suggested we all step back, especially me. I complied reluctantly and watched as Andy struck up a conversation with the man from a safe distance, then convinced him to drop the construction material and drink some juice. Our patient got better and I got smarter.

Being Unspectacularly Effective

EMS is more about avoiding battles than winning them. Leaders who respond to conflict with ego-driven defiance risk lives and compromise their reputations. Often, the best way to maintain authority is to demonstrate it as little as possible.

From scene size-up to departure, priorities should be safety and assessment—neither of which I paid much attention to on that diabetic call until Andy showed up. I was more focused on disarming our patient than on safer alternatives. I felt personally challenged and thought the best way to protect myself and my crew from our patient's aggressive stance was with force. I'm not sure why; maybe I'd watched too many John Wayne movies as a kid. All I know is, the idea of deescalating tension with patience and pleasant conversation, as Andy did, hadn't occurred to me.

Getting the job done on scene in a way that works for everyone is difficult to teach. Classroom exercises often fall short of portraying real-world decision points, such as when and how to engage safely with patients. Even experienced providers can benefit by examining their potential weaknesses as leaders.

Leading Questions

Forget about medicine for a moment; think about your coworkers. Pick one with whom you've worked in the field recently, then ask yourself these questions about that partner's performance:

Can he subordinate his ego to the job? EMS teaches us to be proactive in the field; to take charge. That doesn't mean we can't also take advice. There's nothing wrong with asking for abridged opinions before making difficult decisions. Considering opposing points of view shows strength of character, not weakness.

Is he missing opportunities to do *less*? This will sound counter-intuitive to some, but I've learned to take pride in shutting up and letting my subordinates make things happen. That process begins with leaders who focus on good outcomes, not on who's responsible for them. It helps to have a bias for delegation. Just enjoy watching your people show how capable they are.

As he leads, does he also serve? What should leaders do while subordinates are working effectively without a ton of oversight? Listen and help. Bring the stretcher. Carry the bags. Revel in a reversal of roles. Be mindful of big-picture objectives, but suppress the urge to speak just for the sake of being heard.

Does he ever succeed by being different? Look for opportunities to constructively deviate from what others expect. During difficult calls, that might mean trying extra hard to show a relaxed demeanor. On non-emergent calls, make a special effort to demonstrate concern for the patient, and consider legitimate underlying causes for what seem to be frivolous complaints.

Can he be the sanest one on scene? The more authority you have, the more responsibly you have to use it. Effective leaders don't succumb to the insanity of the moment—quite the opposite. They see themselves as possibly the only unbroken link between hostility and civility.

Does he ever stop setting good examples? Good leadership is about doing all the above, always. If even one of your people try the same techniques when it's their turn to lead, you've accomplished something lasting and exceptional.

Now turn the above questions inward: How do you think you compare to your partner? It's not a contest—just a way to make your self-evaluation a little easier.

As I went through that exercise just now, I realized I've changed a lot since 1995. Although I still have to remind myself at times to say less, listen more, and not take opposition personally, I'm much more aware of my responsibilities to others and am determined to keep coolest when conflicts heat up.

Thanks, Andy.

A HIRE PRIORITY

2015

Ny first job interview went something like this:

> "So, you're . . . Mike? The one who called? When can you start?"

Before you think bad thoughts about some desperate EMS agency, I should mention I was 16 years old and looking for work as an usher in a movie theater.

So maybe movie houses didn't go out of their way to vet unskilled labor when I was a teenager. I'd like to think today's paramedics and EMTs find jobs only after much more thorough evaluations, but I don't know if that's true. What I do know is that although the consequences of hiring a rude ticket-taker are nowhere near as severe as employing an incompetent caregiver, most good interviewing practices aren't industry-specific; they're broad enough to apply to almost any help-wanted scenario.

In this article, we'll discuss some of those practices from the employer's perspective. There's intrigue and gamesmanship on both sides of the desk, but after 41 years as interviewer and interviewee, I'd rather be the one asking the questions.

Interview Basics

What are you looking for in an employee? Wisdom? Honesty? Technical proficiency? It's pretty hard to judge those qualities in a person sitting across from you for 15 minutes.

Try this exercise: Think about your current employees or some other group of workers you know well. Pick one trait that applies to the best of them.

Are they the smartest? The bravest? The nicest? The most experienced? I didn't have to think very long about my answer: My best workers made my job easier. They might not have been the brightest or even the most capable, but each of them found ways to make my life less complicated by grasping the implicit contract between boss and employee: *I do for you and you do for me.*

I'm not claiming managers and their subordinates routinely follow that principle. I've worked for several firms where the corporate rules of engagement were more like, *you do for me because you have to,* or simply, *I do for me.* It takes an innovative company and exceptional people to own the part about helping each other, not merely for altruistic reasons, but because unselfishness and trust are essential elements of good business.

I don't know if you work for a truly innovative employer; probably not—they're pretty rare. I bet your company is looking for exceptional people, though. Distinguishing them from the largely unexceptional majority and, more problematically, from the ones who lack substance but can charm their way through 15 minutes of dialogue, is the primary goal of an employee interview.

Desirable Traits

So how do we cull good candidates from the not-so-good ones?

Remember, the good ones understand the implicit boss/employee contract and will make your job easier. What "raw materials" do they need for that? Reliability, maturity, adaptability, and good judgment are my picks.

Those attributes are qualitative and, therefore, hard to measure, so how many of them can we hope to evaluate during a brief interview?

All of them. Let's run through the list:

Reliability
Detecting this fundamental trait has the highest priority. Even the smartest, most talented people are of no value if they don't show up for work.

- **Good signs:** Applicants who aren't just on time for their interviews; they're early. It's their responsibility—not yours—to allow for traffic, weather, and wardrobe emergencies.

- **Bad signs:** Prospective employees who arrive even one minute late.

Maturity

Beginning with grooming and dress and continuing with behavior during the interview, maturity is the easiest of the four key traits to judge. Whatever a candidate does to make you feel uncomfortable would probably affect patients the same way.

- **Good signs:** Neat business attire complemented by conservative grooming. Even inexperienced interviewees should know the difference between having rights of self-expression, such as extensive tattoos or piercings, and exercising those rights.
- **Bad signs:** Questions asked by applicants in advance about how to get there, what to wear, or whether to bring a résumé; questions asked early in the interview about vacation or sick time; questions asked anytime about drug testing.

Adaptability

I'm going to assume, without a shred of evidence, that most candidates don't enjoy job interviews. I say that because the majority of prospective employees I've met seemed at least mildly uncomfortable before, during, and even after that process. Some were beyond uncomfortable and on their way to non-functional.

A little nervousness isn't a bad thing. Even on the job, controllable anxiety means we care about our performance.

Some of my interviewees confessed their nervousness to me during interviews. Many of them found ways to impress me despite their discomfort. They adapted to unexpected questions and overcame their distress.

A 2005 study by the U.S. Army found that an important trait linked to adaptability is willingness to learn. I'd rather manage people with a realistic sense of what they don't know and an eagerness to improve than those who labor to project invincibility.

- **Good signs:** A candidate's pleasant, constructive affect and cogent replies to unpredictable questions, despite ordinary anxiety.
- **Bad signs:** Anyone who appears overwhelmed during their interview.

Good judgment

One could argue that reliability, maturity, and adaptability are elements of good judgment, but I look at that relationship in reverse: Good judgment, I believe, precedes reliability, maturity, and adaptability on the developmental scale and is the mortar that binds those building blocks of character.

- **Good signs:** Interviewees who answer whatever they're asked with a minimum of editorializing and digression.
- **Bad signs:** Almost anything from a candidate that you wouldn't have said.

High-Frequency Listening

A fundamental interview strategy is to encourage prospective employees to reveal their strengths and weaknesses without them knowing that's the plan. Success depends on establishing a feedback loop, whereby interviewers evaluate candidates' verbal and non-verbal responses, vector toward provocative issues, then immediately pose related questions. Such "high-frequency listening" and real-time follow-up is harder than it sounds. Consider these essentials:

Minimize distractions

The way we used to do this is have someone in the office answer our phones and take messages. That sounds laughably antiquated now, but you can still separate yourself from your smartphone, can't you? Or at least mute it and ignore it? Maybe not. The problem is that frequent interruptions are going to interfere with your focus and signal interviewees—especially the ones worth hiring—that you're either disorganized or rude.

Add a little atmosphere

I liked to evaluate people as they responded to opposite circumstances: at ease and stressed.

Relaxed candidates were more likely to say something revealing about themselves—the kinds of unusual beliefs or values that might come out during collegial conversations. Sometimes, I heard about personal biases or frustrations with past bosses that I considered deal-breakers.

A sympathetic affect can help interviewers encourage sometimes-startling statements from prospective employees. You don't have to explicitly agree; just project a pleasant willingness to listen. Such tactics sound disingenuous, but ferreting out negatives is your responsibility and is much more important than eliciting self-serving positives.

Adding mild-to-moderate stressors to an interview can simulate some challenges candidates would face on the job. For example, multiple concurrent questioners can make it hard for interviewees to formulate answers cautiously. EMS providers who can't process simultaneous sources of input probably aren't the ones you want to hire.

Don't just listen; watch

Deciphering body language is an art beyond the scope of this article, but non-verbal responses are important ways to derive a more complete picture of prospective employees. Let's stick to a few common-sense considerations:

Is eye contact steady enough so you don't feel deceived, but not so riveting that the candidate seems possessed? Is their sweat level appropriate for mild anxiety, not triathlon training? Do they suddenly cross their arms—perhaps indicating defiance—when you ask a difficult question?

The bottom line, I think, for those of us lacking expertise in body language, is whether the applicant's non-verbal behavior makes us uncomfortable.

Processing first impressions

Our initial opinions of people are often valid, but that doesn't mean we shouldn't allow interviewees a moment to adjust before we start making irreversible decisions about their futures. Just keep in mind that the behavior you're seeing is the *best* those candidates can manage.

Preparation

Even with high-frequency listening, you're going to want a question bank you can draw from whenever an interview thread has run its course. I used to bring 5–10 conversation starters to each session.

Avoid common queries that aren't directly related to the job like, "What do you want to do 10 years from now?" Candidates have probably heard that one before.

Consider problem-solving questions based on EMS scenarios. Also, try prompting a reaction to a controversial event or point of view; for example, "Did you hear about the medic who dumped his patient off the stretcher?" If you ask that with a smile or even a chuckle, you might be surprised at the sympathy for aberrant behavior you elicit. Better to learn about that before making an offer.

Instead of waiting for references, ask prospective employees for permission to contact former supervisors. You probably don't need to pursue applicants who decline.

Remember, your goal is to mine nuggets about candidates' character traits; not to facilitate their recitation of practiced rhetoric. Be professional, be thorough, and be opportunistic.

References

Mueller-Hanson, Rose A., Susan S. White, David W. Dorsey, and Elaine D. Pulakos. "Training adaptable leaders: Lessons from research and practice." *U.S. Army Research Institute for the Behavioral and Social Sciences*, 1844 (2005): 5..

Goman, Carol Kinsey. "Busting 5 body language myths." Last modified July 24, 2012. https://www.forbes.com/sites/carolkinseygoman/2012/07/24/busting-5-body-language-myths/?sh=2c5fa6513922.

THE WRITE STUFF

Let's Be Clear

2018

Since writing is communication, clarity can only be a virtue.

—Strunk & White, *The Elements of Style.*

Let me show you the first paragraph of an article I submitted to an EMS publication many years ago. See if you can guess the topic:

> I think I've found an alternative to middle-of-the-night pages, big-boned patients, and interoffice politics: retirement. I've been experimenting with it for three months, as I wait for the therapeutic climate and healing waters of Millersville, Tennessee to kick in.

Was I writing about retirement? Sounds that way, but no. The wonders of Millersville, Tennessee? Wrong again. Here's the next paragraph:

> The biggest challenge has been staying busy. The last time I was this idle, Johnson was President. No, not Andrew Johnson, but thanks for buying into the whole sage-advice-from-a-senior-medic theme.

There's that retirement vibe again, with a lame attempt at humor—neither of which helps you, dear reader, figure out what the heck I was trying to say.

Craving Clarity

I was hoping to write about the EMS version of Trivial Pursuit, a game I'd helped develop, but I seemed more interested in dazzling readers with a pretentious preamble. It's hard to find an audience willing to wade through that much flotsam before knowing the author's intent. By the second paragraph, I needed to be more specific.

You're probably as surprised at my subject as my editor was. She insisted I demystify my topic or pick another. We decided on the latter because I couldn't think of a way to make my story as interesting to others as it was to me. What had once seemed like a compelling narrative had become an example of self-indulgence.

Perhaps you've had a similar problem clarifying a pet theme. Before you waste as much time as I did on a stillborn project, ask yourself if you're getting sidetracked by any of these issues:

Passion

Passion can blind us to life's gray areas and is a poor substitute for diligence, especially when we're crafting technical articles. Left unchecked, passion can also become an unwelcome surrogate for value. A manuscript without value is nothing more than an intellectual exercise for the author and a waste of time for the reader.

Many of us in EMS are passionate about our industry. I think anyone who hears me talk about EMS for more than 10 seconds can tell I have strong feelings about this business. And why wouldn't I? I devoted 20 years of my life to patient care. It was frustrating at times, and even scary, but there were enough rewarding moments to make me feel good about the job most days.

Frustration, fear, exhilaration—these are intense emotions that influence the way we tell stories and the stories we tell. We expect feelings to prompt a writer's point of view, but they can also overwhelm objectivity and lead to arrogant essays filled with opinions masquerading as facts. Sweeping generalizations are one indication of that.

When you write, do you use unconditional terms like *always* or *never*? What about phrases like *there's no question, without a doubt,* or *the truth is*? Such absolutes often exist only in the mind of the author.

Wait, take another look at that last sentence: Can you find the one word that lends flexibility to my comment? *Often,* like *occasionally* and *sometimes*, is a fairly safe way to tame hyperbole. If I'd left out *often*, I'd be refuting every instance of categorical expressions—an exaggeration I wouldn't want to own. According to Strunk & White, "A single overstatement, wherever or however it occurs, diminishes the whole."

The absence of a clear theme—as in my aborted tale of Trivial Pursuit—is another sign of passion overload. So is an unsupported argument weakened further by emotion. Here's one from another author:

> The sad truth of the matter is that some of us have lost the ability to perform an actual hand-on assessment (if we ever really knew how) as skill is replaced by technology. If diagnosis is really 90% of treatment, we're in big trouble, and so are our patients.

Whose "sad truth" is this? What are examples of "hands-on" assessment skills replaced by technology? Who says diagnosis is "90% of treatment"? And what's with that parenthetical implication that we never really knew how to assess?

As a reader, instead of finding anything of value in that excerpt, I'm left wondering whether the author knows what he's talking about.

Elitism

Writers who are elitists (not elite writers) think their knowledge, alone, is reason enough for us not-so-elite readers to appreciate their work. Elitists also believe their experience is as trustworthy as any research, and research at odds with their own opinions is necessarily flawed.

The editorials that elitists offer as scholarly work often feature poor attempts at humor or sarcasm. The onus is on readers to get the jokes. An elitist rendered pliable by a scopolamine drip would probably admit, "I think I'm the cleverest one in the room."

What effect do elitists have on literature? They complicate it. They short-cut explanations of things their minions might not understand. They use bigger words when smaller ones would do. They cram unnecessary detail into paragraphs that should be sentences.

Why do elitists do these things? Because they can.

I should add that most of us who write for a living are way too insecure to be elitists.

Naiveté

I've reviewed dozens of manuscripts by unpublished writers—unpublished outside of casual venues like blogs and social media, that is. Most of those writers seem to underestimate what's required to get their work past traditional publishing's gatekeepers—professional editors, who know the difference between well-intentioned authors and proficient ones.

I can relate to naiveté. I used to think I could be a musician. After experimenting with the clarinet, saxophone, and oboe in high school, I bought one of those early electronic keyboards, taught myself to play, and impressed a bunch of people: my mother, father, and brothers. It wasn't until I worked with real musicians many years later that I realized how clumsy I was compared to the pros. I'd had no idea what it takes to play music for money.

It's hard to blame prospective authors for not appreciating their weaknesses when there's so much unsupervised self-publishing. Rarely do online "friends" criticize ponderous writing. If you want to make written composition more than a hobby, understand that communicating clearly and convincingly takes practice. Some areas to target are:

- **Clichés and colloquialisms.** Not all of your readers grew up speaking English the way you do, and some of them are too young to spot decades-old cultural references. More on that later.
- **Poor or inappropriate analogies.** Straightforward comparisons that help make a point are fine, but don't get too creative. Hint: Likening anyone to Hitler or anything to Armageddon probably won't enhance your credibility with readers.
- **Contradictions and ambiguities.** These might be hard to notice, which is one reason I review my work, like, 17 times. Try reading your manuscript aloud to yourself or give it to someone honest and close to examine. As rock-star novelist Stephen King points out in *On Writing*, if you find yourself deflecting a faithful truth-teller's criticism with "Yes, but . . . ," your piece needs work.

Indifference

Inappropriate or insufficient reinforcement can turn a naïve writer into an apathetic one. In today's open-access publishing environment, where anyone with an Internet connection can self-identify as an artist and get instant gratification via a paroxysm of likes, it's hard for inexperienced authors to find really useful feedback. Consequently, novice writers who don't know any better become indifferent to the creative process, mimic lazy authors, and start embracing some pretty unrealistic notions about high-quality composition, such as:

- **It's like writing a long Facebook post.** You mean except for planning, research, organization, editing, style, syntax, grammar, and punctuation?
- **I should be able to knock this out in an hour or two.** Only if a minute or two of readers' attention is all you want.
- **The editor will fix whatever needs fixing.** Once. Maybe.

One characteristic that seems to be shared by passionate, elitist, naïve, and indifferent writers is a desire to "tell it like it is," as if such noble intent excuses lack of clarity. To the contrary, "tellers" should pamper their readers with unpretentious, unambiguous content. "Clutter is the disease of American writing," says William Zinsser, author of *On Writing Well.* "We are a society struggling with unnecessary words, circular constructions, pompous frills, and meaningless jargon."

If you're as determined as I am to avoid such confusion, maybe your manuscript needs a fresh start. Begin with an opening that's neither dull nor mysterious.

"What's It All About, Alfie?"

When Dionne Warwick first sang that verse in 1966, there weren't any EMS books or magazines. EMTs wouldn't even exist for another three years. Half a century later, though, over 800,000 EMS providers in the U.S. stay current with the help of industry-specific literature. The best of it withstands the scrutiny of those gatekeepers I mentioned above.

What kind of writer are you? Can you dedicate yourself to clear, concise prose in support of a worthwhile theme?

Publishable pieces need beginnings that introduce topics promptly and unequivocally. I'm not suggesting something as tedious as "Today

I will write about oxygen," but rather a few sentences that engage readers and make them want to see more. Let's look at an example:

> Writing for publication can be fulfilling and even cathartic for EMS providers. Having a story to tell is just part of the process; to entice editors, prospective authors must offer clear, persuasive content. Ambiguous, narcissistic prose confuses readers and has little chance of being accepted.

That's the first paragraph of my email to the publisher proposing the article you're reading now. It's just another bit of text by an author trying to make a point: I want to write about writing.

Notice how the reference to EMS in the first sentence implies industry-specific relevance. Without that, the opening paragraph would sound more general and less persuasive. Also, I tried to stimulate interest and show confidence in my topic with strong adjectives like *cathartic* and *narcissistic*.

My work was far from finished, though. Most immediately, it needed a nudge in a practical direction—an indication of more payback for readers than mere opinions I might have about writing.

Something of Value
Here's my second paragraph:

> The proposed piece would focus on style, key story elements, and practical structure. I'd include samples from my own submissions—failures as well as successes—to help illustrate effective manuscript construction. The tone would be conversational.

I'm trying to add value with a "reveal" that taps into my specialized knowledge. I'm suggesting I could write from an unusual or even unique perspective. We have to offer readers something useful in exchange for their discretionary time. Education? Entertainment? Either helps sustain interest.

Although my proposal was a lot shorter than the article it became, there was just as much need for clarity and value. Even compositions as brief and informal as social-media posts would be more persuasive if their authors offered more than ambiguous outrage. Most readers aren't going to waste time deep diving through muddied references.

According to Zinsser, the average reader has an attention span of about 30 seconds. At a high-comprehension reading speed of, say, 150 words per minute, we'd have only as much text as my two paragraphs to draw an audience. That's not much of a challenge for a good storyteller with great material, but medical literature includes many bland, technical topics that are hard to hype. I mean, how are you supposed to turn a piece about COPD into something inspiring?

Let's see what happened when I tried bringing clarity and value to one of the most boring subjects in the world.

The Math Problem

Is there anything more mind-numbing than drug math? I don't think so. Nevertheless, I tackled that topic in a 2012 article. The challenge was to write about drug math in a way that

1. encouraged my audience to stay tuned past the first paragraph, and
2. offered enough value so that readers who did stick around wouldn't feel they'd wasted their time.

My first attempt at an opening was pretty bad, starting with the second paragraph:

> I could begin by telling you about famous people who've had just as much trouble as you with drug math. Okay, I don't really know that, but if it were true, here's what some celebrities might have said:
>
> - "I put 3cc of albuterol in that nebulizer, but I didn't inhale." —Bill Clinton

- "Take my infusion pump. Please." —Henny Youngman
- "Hey kids, can you say, 'administration set'? I knew you could." —Fred (Mr.) Rogers
- "Probably useful, definitely frustrating." —The authors of ACLS
- "Fascinating." —Star Trek's Mr. Spock, the only one who'd enjoy drug math

Remember my earlier point about avoiding obscure cultural references? That's what those hypothetical quotes from Henny Youngman, Fred Rogers, and Mr. Spock would have been for some. Even readers who'd heard of those people wouldn't necessarily have known what they were famous for. I mean, what are the chances a random, millennial EMT ever saw Henny Youngman perform? The guy's been dead for 20 years.

Regarding value, the way I originally expressed formulas in the examples I provided was unnecessarily puzzling. Here's an example of an IV drip-rate calculation:

$$(2\text{mg/min}/4\text{mg/cc}) \times 60\text{gtts/cc} = 30\text{gtts/min}$$

Remember, this is an article aimed at medics having trouble with basic algebra. I don't think I would have done them any favors if I'd left that line alone. All those slashes and abbreviations camouflage the elegance of some straightforward arithmetic.

Sometimes, simple changes in punctuation add clarity. After inserting tactical spaces and a layer of brackets, my formula was less intimidating:

$$([2 \text{ mg/min}] / [4 \text{ mg/cc}]) \times 60 \text{ gtts/cc} = 30 \text{ gtts/min}$$

Prose without enough periods and commas can be just as confusing. Here's an extreme example from one of my writing presentations:

That that is is that that is not is not is that it it is.

Rarely does anyone in the crowd make sense of that. Add a little punctuation, though, and it becomes an indisputable truth:

That that is, is. That that is not, is not. Is that it? It is.

Remember that the next time you're wondering whether punctuation matters.

Struggling Writers: Is There Another Kind?

On days when I felt overwhelmed by EMS, I'd remind myself patient care isn't supposed to be easy. Neither is writing.

"Writing for most is laborious and slow," say William Strunk and E.B. White, whose *Elements of Style* is perhaps the single most practical tool for writers of all pedigrees.

"Writing is hard, even for authors who do it all the time," echoes essayist Roger Angell.

But the most useful lesson I can leave you with—one that summarizes our theme and suggests a realistic next step—is from Professor Zinsser:

> Writers must constantly ask: What am I trying to say?
> Then they must look at what they've written and ask:
> Have I said it?

References

King, Stephen. *On Writing*. New York: Scribner, 2000.

Zinsser, William. *On Writing Well, Seventh Edition*. New York: HarperCollins, 2006.

Strunk, William, Jr., and E. B. White. *The Elements of Style*. 4th ed. New York: Allyn and Bacon, 2000.

Brewer, E. Cobham. *Brewer's Dictionary of Phrase & Fable*. 18th Edition. New York: Harper, 2009.

Author's Note

Don't underestimate the consequences of poorly written casual correspondence—e.g., emails, social-media posts, and tweets. They can be even more harmful to your reputation than verbal gaffes because they float around the Internet indefinitely. Get in the habit of taking another look at whatever you're about to send.

SELF-EMPLOYMENT

2017

"Headquarters to Mike's Ambulance."
"Mike's Ambulance—go ahead."
"Hey Mike, could you respond to the diff breather at
741 Broadway?"
"Sure. Is that credit or debit?"
"Credit—the card you have on file."
"Ok, no problem. So, one diff breather at 741
Broadway. Anything else?"
"Nah, not right now. You're the best. Talk to ya later."

That's my notion of the ideal job: me and my hand-picked partner answering prepaid 9-1-1 calls on *my* ambulance. No corporate politics, no micromanaging by administrators, no committees tasked with token projects. I'd work the way I wanted, pay myself fairly, and even take naps when I wasn't busy.

If only it were that simple.

Self-employment is enticing if you're tired of reporting to someone else. Daily reminders of not being in charge—abrasive bosses, subjective evaluations, and silly rules—can be more stressful than patient care itself. But full-time self-employment is relatively uncommon in the U.S., accounting for only about 10% of the workforce. To borrow an old saying, if it were easy, more people would do it.

During 33 consecutive years of running my own show at least some of the time, I've been able to chart a course around most workplace indignities, but not without other impediments sole proprietors know best: irregular paychecks, extra taxes, long hours, continuous record-keeping and, most notably, finding and keeping customers. To succeed on your own, you need to be not only the best boss, but also the ideal employee: courteous, conscientious, and competent.

If you're considering self-employment, even as a sideline to supplement EMS earnings, this article will either help you get started or warn you away.

Paying the Price for Independence

You might be surprised at how many opportunities there are for EMS providers to make extra money as independent contractors. Writing, teaching, and working special events are common ways in our industry of supplementing income through self-employment, but getting such jobs can be easier than understanding the ongoing administrative effort they require. I'm going to break that down for you after defining what it means to be your own boss—as far as the feds are concerned, at least.

The IRS says you're self-employed if you do business as a sole proprietor, independent contractor, or member of a partnership. A partnership would be an unusual arrangement for an EMS provider, even for side work, so let's focus on sole proprietors and independent contractors—two terms that are almost synonymous for people who run their own businesses.

"Sole proprietor" implies a single owner/employee of an unincorporated company that can sell either goods or services, while independent contractors usually are service providers who may have employees other than themselves, but often don't. Either title fits me—an unincorporated service provider with no employees other than myself. More importantly, from the IRS's point of view, I get to decide what work I'll do and how I'll do it. That makes me independent—a significant distinction because taxes imposed on such workers are calculated differently than they are for employees. For example, most employees pay 7.65% for FICA (Social Security plus Medicare) while independent contractors owe almost double that. An extra 7% of, say, $40,000 in net earnings comes to $2,800 a year—not a pleasant prospect for the self-employed.

(I'm going to use the abbreviated term "contractor" to mean either "independent contractor" or "sole proprietor"; that is, a worker who meets IRS criteria for independence.)

What if you want to keep your primary job as an employee of an EMS agency *and* earn extra money as a contractor—e.g., combine your situation with mine? You're still going to pay that extra FICA burden known as self-employment taxes on your self-employment income. And that's not the only way your world will change when you work for yourself. Let me highlight some of those other differences, beginning with how my compensation as a full-time self-employed person likely differs from most of yours as employees.

Income

My checks come from customers, not employers. Sometimes I see a dollar amount much bigger than what I used to make in the field, partly because there's nothing withheld for taxes, FICA, retirement, or health insurance, but then I remember I still have to pay for those things.

Oh, and just because I got a check today doesn't mean I'll get another in a week, a month, or ever, because (1) I may not be hired again, and (2) even if I am, my customer might not pay me. More on the difference between money owed, billed, and collected later.

For most of you, self-employment wouldn't be your main source of income; you're employees of EMS agencies and, as such, have funds withheld from your regular wages for FICA and income taxes. Those deductions from your paychecks won't cover what you'll owe on self-employed income, though; you'll have to increase the amount withheld by your employer via a revised W-4 form and/or pay quarterly estimated taxes using IRS Form 1040-ES. Failure to do either would likely leave you with unpaid taxes and perhaps penalties at the end of the year.

Expenses

Here's another catch about making money as a contractor: To be realistic about what you're earning, you first have to deduct related expenses from whatever you're paid. Sometimes those expenses are almost equal to, or even greater than, your income, which means you're not really making any money at all.

Suppose I'm promised $1,000 for a 60-minute conference presentation. Sounds good, right? Maybe not. Here's why:

- I might have to pay travel expenses out of pocket. Even if the conference is within driving distance, I could be responsible for gas, depreciation on my car, lodging, and meals.
- The time I spend preparing my presentation and traveling to and from the conference is worth something; how much is somewhat arbitrary and tends to be set by the market. The more people there are who do what I do, the less I'll be able to charge. After expenses are factored in, my $1,000 fee may or may not cover all of my time. It depends on how much I think I deserve and how much less than that I'm willing to accept. Is $20 per hour too little? Is $75 per hour a windfall? Should I insist on what I think I'm worth or take what I can get?
- My biggest expense of all might be taxes. Even if my client reimburses me for travel, I'll still have to pay both the employer's and the employee's share of FICA plus income tax on my net fee. That could be $250 or more—15% for FICA plus 10% of $1,000 if I'm in the lowest income tax bracket.

On the positive side, it's much easier for contractors like me to reduce taxes by deducting work-related expenses against income. I routinely decrease my taxable income legitimately by subtracting anything and everything related to earning my pay. Supplies, office expenses, utilities, insurance, publications, repairs, rent, advertising, travel, lodging, professional services—anything I spend that contributes to my income gets deducted before I calculate what I owe Uncle Sam.

Beginning with tax year 2018, it's even more advantageous to be a contractor. I can deduct an extra 20% of my self-employed net income, but employees are no longer allowed to deduct most unreimbursed business expenses.

Self-Employment: A Lifestyle as Much as an Occupation

Say you decide to start a side business teaching CPR. You get certified as an instructor, maybe print some business cards, put the word out, and then . . . what? Sit back and wait for the phone to ring?

Not if you're serious about getting paid by anyone other than family members.

Running a business—even a small one—is a curious mix of big-picture preparation and attention to detail. It requires so much more than a good idea. Of the 30-plus people I've known who got as far as advertising their new ventures, perhaps five or six made enough money to cover the cost of their stationery. I think the main reason for such a low success rate is one basic misunderstanding about running a small business: It's not just an occupation; it's a lifestyle. Eight-hour days, five-day work weeks, and two-week vacations—practices common in corporations—are fantasies for me and most of the contractors I know. It's not that our work is incredibly hard or unsatisfying; it's just that bosses of one-person companies don't get to delegate anything.

In my experience, cultivating customers is the most important and least predictable part of a contractor's job. Clients with business questions are going to expect the same extended evening and weekend hours they get from bigger firms. The ones who know that your home is your office might even call long after most nine-to-five employees have gone to bed. You can turn off the phone and tell yourself you're entitled to as much quiet time as anyone else, but being relentlessly available to your customers is one of the best ways to distinguish yourself from your competition. I have taken 2 AM telephone calls from clients who haven't even been sober.

Here are other make-or-break aspects of self-employment.

Exposure

When I took on my first clients as a part-time "computer tutor" and software developer in the '80s, the most widespread social media were letters and telephones. A contractor's rudeness or bad grammar might undo a deal, but damage was likely limited to one lead.

Today, every public post on electronic media carries a risk of establishing or contributing to an unfavorable reputation throughout your market. It's a problem that should be easy to avoid by suppressing the urge to behave badly in print, but for many, the right to say pretty much anything trumps the wisdom of doing so.

Teaching, writing, and speaking at conferences are safer, more constructive ways of getting known.

Customer service

Finding customers is hard, but keeping them can be even harder. It's not enough to identify their needs; you must demonstrate that understanding by showing your passion for quality and service every day. I'm using the word "passion" because I can't think of a better way to express the uncompromising devotion to customers you're going to need.

Think about what *you* dislike about being a customer. Unreliability of goods and services would be near the top of my list. I hate when I pay for promises that aren't kept. Even worse is when I can't find someone to fix a problem. Don't be the kind of businessperson that forgets who is supposed to serve whom.

Billing and collecting

Business relationships begin with willing buyers and sellers; however, deriving revenue from a sale requires more than a customer's stated or even written agreement to pay. The process of collection usually starts with an invoice: a document confirming who bought what from you, at what price, and when you should be paid.

I'm amazed at how long it takes some contractors to generate invoices for services rendered. I can't think of any administrative activities other than customer service that should take priority over billing. And following up on collection is just as important. There's a name for contractors who do neither: hobbyists.

Recordkeeping

Sometimes I'll hear a colleague boast of a business that "runs itself." That's about as realistic as a self-cleaning ambulance. Even if you're blessed with an opportunity to earn passive income—royalties for original work, perhaps—you still have to keep track of revenue and expenses or pay someone to do that for you.

Simple bookkeeping doesn't require a CPA; just comfort with arithmetic and a willingness to learn accounting basics. It isn't as hard as you might think, thanks to state-of-the-art software.

When I started my company, I used an entry-level accounting program to help familiarize myself with no-frills bookkeeping. Later, I switched to a spreadsheet I developed for myself. You can even use pencil and paper if you like; just understand what details you'll be expected to report at tax time. Begin by reviewing Schedule C, "Profit or Loss from Business," which gets attached to IRS Form 1040.

Thrift

Speaking of profit, if you're not showing one, consider the following:

- Are you spending money you haven't earned? Buying fancy office furnishings or paying yourself a salary instead of investing those funds in your business are common mistakes.
- Are you renting space when you could work out of your home? Spare bedrooms are the only headquarters I've ever had as a contractor.

You don't have to pretend to be bigger than you are. Customers respect service more than size and would much rather speak with you than some assistant.

Next Steps

What's a good starting point for anyone contemplating self-employment? Talk to others who've done it. If it feels right, start small. Define your business. Spend a few hours a week preparing, then a couple of hours a day courting clients.

Pursue opportunities head on. Work for little or nothing at first, just to build credibility and gain experience. Get used to marketing yourself, but don't even think about leaving your day job until you have paying customers, and even then, only if you crave independence more than security. Develop a reputation for excellence one customer at a time.

Being your own boss isn't about wealth or privilege; it's mostly about having enough independence to treat others the way you want to be treated. That alone makes me happier.

References

Hipple, Steven F. and Laurel A. Hammond. "Self-employment in the United States." U.S. Bureau of Labor Statistics. *Spotlight on Statistics*, March 2016.

Internal Revenue Service. "Self-Employed Individuals Tax Center." Updated December 7, 2016. https://www.irs.gov/businesses/small-businesses-self-employed/self-employed-individuals-tax-center.

Author's Note

It's as risky to write about income tax reporting rules as it is to quote ACLS guidelines. Both seem to change every few years. I updated this piece to be consistent with 2018-2019 laws, which gave contractors a few extra advantages over employees.

ENOUGH STUFF
Inventory Management in EMS

2016

You're back in quarters after an asymptomatic cardiac patient refuses transport. You finish your PCR, attach a copy of the precautionary rhythm strip, then head to the supply closet for a fresh pack of electrodes.

The bin is empty. Before you have a chance to start a scavenger hunt, another call comes in. With no electrodes left in your vehicle, you grab the only set from another ambulance and make a mental note to ration EKGs the rest of your shift.

Material control is hardly a glamorous topic. I've never seen a movie or television show about tracking inventory (reality-TV producers, take note), and I don't remember Johnny or Roy ever saying, "Ah, Rampart, negative on that IV, we're out of needles," but stocking adequate quantities of mission-critical items in EMS is just as important as maintaining vehicles or hiring people to staff them. Each of those tasks requires planning and is usually undervalued until it's not done.

What, then, should EMS providers know about inventory control?

Inventory Management Basics

Inventory is a collective term for stored goods—not only saleable products like cars and trucks, but also tires, spark plugs, steering wheels, and other components needed to build those vehicles. We don't manufacture products in EMS, so we'll focus on buying instead of building.

Say you purchase nonrebreather masks: When you pay that invoice, you lose the option to use those funds for other supplies or for income-producing investments. That "time value of money" used to be a big factor in inventory decisions, but with interest rates still low, "borrowing" cash from yourself is relatively cheap.

That doesn't mean inventory costs nothing to keep. You still have to store it, move it, track it, and throw it out when it expires. An even bigger factor is having enough stock to service your customers; or, in the case of EMS, to care for your patients.

In the corporate world, we talk about "lost-opportunity costs" as penalties for running out of products. The opportunity we're losing is almost always selling more.

In EMS, lost opportunities to treat people due to missing or expired supplies can carry much more severe consequences than lower revenues. EMS providers need to protect themselves and their patients by embracing inventory control as a well-documented business practice with high stakes in the essential services.

So what can we learn from the ways other industries keep track of their stuff?

Push or Pull?

There are two fundamental approaches to managing materials: "push" systems, most of which are derivatives of something called *material requirements planning* (MRP), and "pull" systems, also known as *just-in-time* (JIT). Both schemes were introduced in the 1960s—MRP in the U.S. and JIT in Japan. Although MRP and JIT have different rules, their goals are the same: minimize inventory costs while maximizing sales of manufactured items. In EMS, the latter objective would be comparable to maximizing preparedness for patient care.

MRP "pushes" component parts—tires, spark plugs, and steering wheels in our automotive example—through factories, based mostly on the following information:

- Sales forecasts of finished goods, such as cars
- Bills of materials, which are "recipes" showing everything needed to make one complete unit

- Available quantities of components and finished goods
- Lead times for buying components to make finished goods

Right away, MRP sounds more complicated than what we need in EMS, where we're just stocking basic items like dressings and drugs purchased wholesale from medical suppliers. There are useful elements of MRP we'll come back to, though.

JIT "pulls" components through factories as needed. Sticking with our car example, when the last spark plug leaves the supply bin, an order is generated for more. That order, in true JIT companies, initiates a purchase of parts from a vendor so close, and so coordinated with the factory, delivery occurs within hours. That level of cooperation between vendors and their customers is difficult to achieve in the U.S., where partnerships between buyers and sellers of goods are harder to establish than in JIT's birthplace, Japan.

So far, neither MRP nor JIT sounds like an ideal system for EMS, but let's see which features of each might help us manage supplies.

MRP versus JIT for EMS

MRP is a sophisticated tool. It considers three important aspects of inventory control: how much you have of each item, how many more finished goods you should build or buy to satisfy demand, and what components you'll need to do that. Even if we ignore that last part about components, MRP can still teach EMS providers a few things:

- Do the best you can to estimate how much of each purchased item you'll need in the coming year.
- Include allowances for expiration, waste, and theft of supplies when forecasting demand.
- Report usage of supplies as it occurs.
- Be able to track and occasionally verify stock at multiple locations.
- Factor lead times and inaccurate usage forecasts into purchase timing and quantities.

Push systems like MRP depend on reasonably accurate sales forecasts in most industries. If you know what you're going to sell, you can calculate what components you'll need to make those items.

EMS is different because we're not manufacturing anything, but still need to estimate how many masks, electrodes, dressings, gloves, etc. we're going to use in the coming year. Ideally, we'd do that based on the expected distribution of presenting problems, then average the supplies needed for each.

For example, we'd need either a nasal cannula or a nonrebreather, a package of electrodes, an IV set, and averaged amounts of oxygen, aspirin, and nitroglycerin for each instance of acute coronary syndrome. We'd multiply the number of expected ACS cases by the quantity of each associated item to get our gross material requirements for that illness.

Here's the problem: I have yet to see reliable, zero-based projections of chief complaints. Plugging inaccurate forecasts or inventory balances into fully automated MRP systems merely makes it possible to screw up at the speed of light. The only way I can think of to estimate demand in EMS is to begin with last year's, then massage it according to known or suspected changes.

JIT is less about forecasting and more about minimizing or even eliminating inventory. It reminds us that close cooperation with vendors is mutually beneficial; suppliers are assured business by customers who want to depend on quick turn-around of purchase orders. JIT's lessons for EMS are:

- Don't buy more material than you need.
- Establish long-term relationships with vendors whenever possible.
- When you notice a shortage, communicate that promptly to further reduce lead times.

What can go wrong? Well, EMS agencies aren't going to house mini branches of suppliers, as some big manufactures do. Anything that gets in the way of immediate response by vendors to customers' needs—bad weather, distance, missed payments, delayed orders—will quickly drive inventory to zero and, therefore, threaten continued operations.

If you're thinking it's so much easier to *talk* about implementing even modified forms of MRP or JIT than to make either happen, you're right. Most EMS agencies don't have enough manpower or broad-based business expertise to babysit such complex initiatives. There's software out there that can help—programs like Operative IQ, with comprehensive inventory-management modules, and ePCR packages that bundle stock-control capabilities with core features. Or you could try this:

An Unsophisticated but Useful Inventory Spreadsheet

If you're looking for a basic material control technique that's easier than manual number crunching, build a spreadsheet with the following columns left to right:

A. **Item:** A short, unique, descriptive term.
B. **Starting Balance:** A physical count of each item at a point in time (you'll reset columns B through H when you take a new count at least once a year).
C. **+ Receipts:** A running sum of quantities received (e.g., 50 + 100 + 25).
D. **Last Receipt:** The date of the most recent delivery, to help track which transactions have already been entered.
E. **– Usage:** A running sum of quantities used. Getting this information from field personnel will be one of your biggest challenges. You'll have to establish a procedure whereby usage of supplies is documented along with other patient-care details.
F. **Last Usage:** The date of most recent usage.
G. **Adjust +/–:** A running sum of corrections for waste, expiration, returns, etc. Most adjustments will be subtractions that should be preceded by minus signs.
H. **Last Adjustment:** The date of the most recent adjustment.
I. **On-Hand Quantity:** Starting balance + receipts – usage + adjustments expressed as a formula (e.g., $=Bn + Cn - En + Gn$, where n is the row number).
J. **On Order:** A running sum of quantities due, adjusted after each delivery.

K. Next Due: The next expected delivery date, if any.

L. Available Quantity: On hand plus on order expressed as a formula (e.g., =In + Jn).

M. Annual Forecast: Expected annual usage, probably estimated from prior usage.

N. Lead Time: The average number of days it takes to restock from the time an item is ordered until it's delivered.

O. Standard Purchase: A reminder of how many units are normally ordered at one time. Such so-called "economic purchase quantities" depend on price breaks, forecast accuracy, and storage space. Calculating them according to all those factors is outside the scope of this article. To keep it simple, order an amount that doesn't take up too much space, won't expire before it's used, and won't often leave you with unanticipated shortages. That's usually a few months' worth.

P. Stock Alert: A formula (=IF(Ln/Mn<Nn/365,"Buy"," ")) that produces a conditional message (*buy*) when the available quantity will be exhausted according to the forecast, before more can be delivered, based on standard lead time.

Q. Comments: Miscellaneous remarks.

You're going to populate the spreadsheet with every item you wish to track, one to a row. You might wish to start with just a few supplies to get an idea of the discipline involved. Later, you could insert a column after ID called *Location* and start tracking inventory movement from and to each station and vehicle.

Adjust column widths and formats as needed. Feel free to make any other changes to the spreadsheet that best fit your agency.

To take material planning further, you'd need a database management system (DBMS) instead of a spreadsheet. DBMS software is much better at tracking the details behind each of those row-and-column entries—histories of inventory transactions, for example. A generic DBMS package like Microsoft Access is the next step up for agencies that don't want to buy a dedicated inventory management program but prefer to develop something more sophisticated than a spreadsheet without needing an IT professional in house.

Homegrown software isn't a solution for everybody; at the very least, you'd need someone on staff who can master DBMS software like Access and has experience managing digital information. If your agency doesn't have such a resource, professionally developed software would be a better option.

The Essence of Inventory Control

Whether you use computers or pencil and paper, the fundamental principles of inventory management are the same:

1. Everyone who touches items you're tracking is accountable for inventory accuracy.
2. Begin by counting everything, then add or subtract every transaction that changes opening balances.
3. The causes of missing or erroneous transactions that lead to incorrect balances and, therefore, jeopardize patient care, need to be whittled down until inventory figures are routinely believable.
4. Forecasts are inherently inaccurate. Keep trying to fine-tune yours.
5. In this time of low inventory carrying costs, it's better to buy more material to take advantage of volume discounts and avoid stock-outs than to test JIT-oriented, razor-thin margins of error.
6. Rule #5 is, of course, limited by expiration dates and storage space. You can help maximize the latter by paying attention to the former.

Conclusion

Inventory management isn't a self-serving administrative exercise; it's an undervalued but strategic element of EMS. Agencies that control their materials improve their chances of offering patients the right care at the right time.

NEGOTIATING
EMS

2016

You're a paramedic dispatched to a middle-aged male complaining of chest pain. When you arrive at the scene, your patient says he's feeling better. He can't or won't characterize the pain and denies cardiac history. He mentions an EKG recorded during a physical last year, but he heard nothing more about it. His disdain for doctors is unmistakable.

You sense his reluctance to be transported or even examined, so you suggest moving to the ambulance, where you know you'll have a better chance to continue care. He refuses. By the time you offer a "quick check" on scene, he's already dismissing you.

The patient is mentating well; you can't treat him against his will. What you can do is negotiate with him. You probably do that a lot with patients. Also with bosses, coworkers, spouses, parents, friends, teachers, salespeople, service providers, doctors, nurses, and sometimes even your kids.

Most of the time, I don't think we're even aware we're negotiating. Maybe that's why we often don't negotiate very well.

Making the Most of Undervalued Techniques

Negotiation isn't a skill we're born with, although some of us who like to think so would no more consider taking lessons in negotiation than in child-rearing. That's too bad, because with a little study and practice, negotiation can become an ally, a business partner, or even a rich uncle who leaves you thousands of dollars. If the idea of saving money and getting people to do what you want interests you, read on.

Are you still there? If so, let me congratulate both of us on a successful negotiation. That's what we've just had, you and I. You're granting me a slice of your discretionary time in return for something you perceive as valuable: this text. I've gained a reader who might buy something from one of the advertisers camped out on this page, thereby making my publisher a little happier with me. It's a win-win outcome—the kind negotiators should seek.

Why Win-Win Is Important

Suppose you're offered a job with East Adipose Ambulance for minimum wage. You ask the boss if you might be able to make a little more than that, but he says, "Hey, I can hire anyone off the street for what I pay you. Take it or leave it!" You reluctantly accept the offer because you have a family and no other income. End of negotiation. Boss 1 Employee 0, right?

Actually, it's more like Boss 0 Employee 0, or even Boss -1 Employee 0, although the folks at East Adipose probably wouldn't realize that. By alienating you not only with the lowest possible offer, but also with disrespect, they're practically guaranteeing whatever money they save on your salary will be more than offset by the cost of your ill will in the future.

It didn't have to go that way. Your boss could have mentioned frequent overtime as an additional source of earnings or agreed to re-evaluate your status in six months. Those aren't magnanimous gestures, but at least they show a willingness to consider your needs.

Negotiating works best when both parties feel they won something. Getting there isn't as hard as you might think.

Know the Balance of Power

When I was growing up, "balance of power" was something scary between the U.S. and the Soviet Union: the ability of one giant country to scorch more earth than the other. Back-channel bargaining kept that from becoming anything more than a hypothetical contest.

For peace-loving individuals like you and me, balance of power means knowing your strengths and weaknesses before negotiating.

Are you the buyer or the seller in a buyers' market or a sellers' market? Do you have something rare and valuable that someone wants, or vice versa? Is there a deadline that has more of an impact on one party than the other?

In our chest-pain case, the patient owns the balance of power. He perceives no advantage to an ED visit and has the right to decline. Unless the medic highlights the elevated risk of sudden death in an imaginative way, there isn't going to be a transport.

Innovation fuels negotiation. In the early 90s, I wanted to buy an inexpensive but very popular car—so popular, there was much more demand than supply. The salesman wasn't going to budge on price until I suggested I might want two cars instead of one. The logic was that my wife's Corolla had become a high-mileage liability—like my car—and would need to be replaced within a year or so anyway.

The unanticipated possibility of two sales commissions and two profitable trade-ins for the dealer swung the balance of power in my favor. I got both cars at substantial discounts.

Don't Let Them Know What You're Thinking

If I'd started my negotiation by admitting how much I wanted that car, I probably wouldn't have gotten any concessions. Why? Because the dealer would have sensed my desperation and just waited me out.

The caregiver in the opening narrative faces a similar situation. He knows an isolated incident of chest pain without history or other risk factors could be benign. He may not be a bigger fan of doctors and hospitals than his patient. However, if he were to verbalize those feelings, he'd put an end to any hope of negotiating transport—a goal arguably best for both patient and provider when chest discomfort is significant enough to require EMS.

To Get, Be Willing To Give

Our medic showed he's willing to compromise by offering an expedited exam on scene. That suggestion didn't solve anything, but maybe it would have if the medic hadn't given up so easily. What if he'd added, "Look, I know you don't want to go to the hospital, and you don't have to. You're calling the shots. I'm only saying I might be able to get you some more information about what caused that pain, and then give you a chance to decide what you want to do."

The medic would be making a concession in his practice primarily to bring about a desirable outcome for himself and his agency, but also to help his patient choose wisely. While it would be cool to catch a life-threatening condition during an abbreviated exam, it's still a win-win if EMS can just document an above-average effort to assess a patient who then makes an informed decision.

Be Willing to Walk Away

Being emotionally vested in a particular outcome is usually a mistake. When I visited that automobile showroom 20-plus years ago, I knew I had to be willing to leave without a new car. Be patient; go home and retool your strategy. Besides, the mere act of walking out may cause the other party to reconsider.

EMS providers recognize limits, too, when negotiating next steps with patients. If our middle-aged male had suggested the medic leave some nitroglycerine in case the pain came back, that would have been a deal-breaker. Sometimes, we have no choice but to walk away knowing it isn't the best outcome for either party.

Negotiation Customs Vary

In some parts of the world, negotiation is much more commonplace than in the U.S. When I was in Mexico in the late 70s, I learned very quickly not to buy anything for more than a few dollars' worth of pesos without negotiating a lower price—sometimes less than half of what was initially asked. However, gaining a few "concessions" didn't make me think for a minute I'd come out ahead in a nation of world-class hagglers.

Even if you live in a region where bargaining is the exception rather than the rule, you can gain significant advantages in the workplace and marketplace just by becoming a more knowledgeable, more effective negotiator. Begin by considering the suggestions in this article. There's no cost or obligation. Now that's a deal!

Author's Note

I can't think of a practical skill that's been more helpful than negotiating in both my business and EMS careers.

SURVIVING PARAMEDIC SCHOOL

2017

What's it like to go to paramedic school? Before I can even think of an answer, I feel catecholamines kick in, as if a preceptor just told me the next tube is mine. Maybe that sounds exciting to some of you, but for me, upgrading from EMT was an unnatural act—scary, hard, and not anything like the seamless exercise I'd imagined. I wasn't even sure it made sense for me to change careers and work full-time in the field.

In my opinion, success in paramedic school has lots to do with expectations: The easier you think it'll be, the more trouble you'll probably have. Not knowing what I was getting into certainly lengthened *my* learning curve. I made the mistake of assuming the curriculum wouldn't be a problem because I'd already earned a degree and thought I had plenty of EMS experience (a whole two years!).

Becoming a paramedic was harder for me than getting my bachelor's degree, mostly because I hated people watching me perform. I hadn't factored those incessant over-the-shoulder evaluations into my expectations. (During four years of engineering school, my practical skills had been graded in only two courses, and one of them was Phys Ed.) I almost quit.

When I became a paramedic instructor, I saw the importance of flexibility among incoming students. The ones who succeeded not only adapted to circumstances much different than they'd expected, but also weren't wedded to erroneous assumptions like these:

1. **I can make room for paramedic school without major changes to my life.** Expect the curriculum to be all-consuming. There's little time for anything else. Explain to your significant other you'll be away a lot and when you're home, you're going to be sleep-deprived, cranky, and preoccupied. Some relationships won't last until graduation.

   a. *Mistake 1A: No reason to cancel that ski trip.* Don't schedule vacations during school; in fact, don't plan any recreational activities. And don't take days off just because you feel like it. It's easier than you think to fall behind, and there won't be any teachers or guidance counselors waiting to help.

   b. *Mistake 1B: Volunteering as often as possible will reinforce what I'm learning.* Volunteering has merit—just not during medic school. Hanging around at the squad may sound like ideal study time, but it hardly ever works out that way. Plus, there's the risk of ending up on a lengthy call and missing class. Don't expect instructors, preceptors, or course directors to excuse lateness or absence because of your service to humanity.

2. **Studying is overrated.** If we exclude the ridiculously gifted among us who understand everything they read or hear the first time, the rest of us need daily repetition and reinforcement. Practical rotations help, but you also have to hit the books and think about what you're learning.

   a. *Mistake 2A: My EMS experience will get me through.* During 11 years on the faculty of a well-known paramedic program, I didn't see any correlation between the number of years students had accumulated in EMS and the likelihood they'd graduate. Even AEMTs who'd already covered some of the ALS material didn't seem to have an advantage.

3. **Healthy habits are nice to have, but not essential.** Eat nutritious meals as often as you can and try to set aside at least six hours a day for sleep—especially before exams. If you're not able to do either, remember sugar is elementary brain food. Tactical candy bars helped me stay alert during more than one test.

4. **Nurses don't know nothin'.** You'll hear this from some medics who think that nurses need step-by-step direction. Do the field of emergency medicine a favor and let that rumor stop

with you. Not only is it untrue, it's demeaning to people who'll be contributing to your evaluations, and an unwise application of free speech. In fact, don't bad-mouth anyone—classmates, teachers, preceptors, administrators. Deal with disagreements in private or not at all.

    a.   *Mistake 4A: Old medics don't remember anything.* Here's what they'll most likely remember: how much of a pain in the ass you were when you tried to impress them with wisdom culled from textbooks.

    b.   *Mistake 4B: Doctors don't know what I know about street medicine.* Correct. They know much more, except maybe the part about chronic back pain.

5. **I paid tuition; they'll make me a medic.** To think of paramedic school as just another service provider would be a gross miscalculation. You, the customer, aren't always right. Unfair things will happen. You won't always understand why you got a test question wrong, why you were criticized, or why some classmates did better than you. Even if you're a good student and a nice person, you'll have to work hard to get by. Your tuition is just another at-risk investment.

The worst mistake you can make in paramedic school is a combination of all the above: failure to adjust to a new reality for the duration of the program. Expect lots of work—much more than you had in high school—and little help. Be flexible, keep an open mind, don't make excuses, and just concentrate on getting the best results you can.

EPILOGUE

Early in 2020, I was driving home with a load of groceries when I noticed flashing red lights a few cars behind me. As I pulled over so an ambulance from an adjacent Tennessee county could pass, I imagined an unstable patient attached to a heart monitor, with oxygen and drugs flowing through plastic tubes to vital organs. I couldn't help it; I've been a paramedic for 26 years.

I won't make it to 30. On February 1, 2023, I'll retire from EMS. That's the plan. I tell myself it's silly to stay in this industry after not practicing medicine since 2013, when I took a leave of absence to recover from my last back injury. I resigned six months later because I still didn't feel confident I could lift, or even bend, as needed. That was a big disappointment for me, but it would have been worse for my patients and partners if I couldn't handle the job's physical demands.

In the eight years since, I've kept my paramedic license current because there's always a chance I'll feel better and return to the field. Sure, and maybe learn to play the harpsichord, too. Enough already.

I'm not complaining. I've had two fulfilling careers: engineering followed by EMS. The former gave me the means to try the latter. It was an unusual move—one that most of my business colleagues wouldn't have understood, had they known. That's why I didn't tell them. One day, I just left. I needed to try something different after two decades as a desk-bound white-collar worker.

EMS, with its character-building successes and failures, turned out to be a good fit. I enjoyed the nervous excitement that helped me focus before each shift. More importantly, I felt proud of what I was: a senior paramedic in a busy 9-1-1 system.

Now I'm faced with losing not just that hard-earned status, but also my identity as a rescuer. I've been that person for so long, it's hard to remember what it felt like to have a "normal" job; to put on a suit instead of a uniform and carry a briefcase instead of a stethoscope; to crunch numbers and attend meetings instead of assessing illnesses and treating trauma; to build information systems and serve large groups of customers rather than focusing on one sick patient at a time.

Being a paramedic has inspired and pleased me more than anything else I've done professionally. There aren't nearly as many life-and-death scenarios in EMS as the public thinks, but when it was my turn to manage a true emergency, I enjoyed the challenge. I already miss the satisfaction of recognizing disease patterns and knowing how to respond. Like most medics, I want to be the one in charge.

So what happens when I leave EMS? The only thing I'll be in charge of is my own well-being. I'm not even sure my cats will need me. They can go feral faster than I can straighten up in the morning. As for my wife, she's usually the adult in the room. Helen needs looking after about as much as Ronda Rousey.

I'm too old and out of date to return to the corporate world unless they need engineers who can birth babies. Then there's my health: I'm not very mobile, but I can think and write. I've also seen terrible things plus a few miracles. Does any of that make me marketable?

All this insecurity is reminding me of my last patient. We'll call him Sam. Neither of us knew I was working my final shift when I saw him lying on his company's cafeteria floor one January afternoon. He was conscious and seemed alert.

I'd treated Sam before. He'd had a stroke as a young man. Partial paralysis was likely a lifelong consequence.

It wasn't unusual for Sam to fall, but this was the first time I'd seen him struggle to get up. Even with one contracted arm and an unsteady gait, he got around pretty well. He was usually friendly and upbeat, but when I found him that day, he was crying.

"Are you hurt?" I asked. He said he didn't think so. I examined him quickly, then helped him into a plastic chair and grabbed one for myself at a table near where he'd fallen. We had most of the dining area to ourselves. Sam wiped his eyes on one sleeve and started talking.

"It gets hard sometimes," he said, as if to justify his emotion. I told him not to worry about that, then waited for him to continue. He did—for 45 minutes.

Sam told me about his stroke, his long rehabilitation, and how far he still was from feeling whole. What I remember most about our conversation is that the longer he spoke, the more he seemed to brighten up. I found that odd. I would have expected his story of incurable, disabling illness to fuel his despair, not lessen it. Yet there he was, sounding more and more optimistic. It was as if he'd rebooted his adaptability.

When it was time for both of us to move along, Sam told me he was ready to go back to work. That was fine with me. I was relieved he didn't need anything more therapeutic than a discreet listener.

It took me many years of caring for strangers to draw wisdom from patients like Sam—the ones whose biggest needs are social, not medical. Despite a paramedic's bias for action, I've learned that sometimes, people just need to talk; to sort through long-standing problems without expecting solutions. My engineering brain thinks that's a waste of time, but engineers don't know everything.

I'm more comfortable writing than talking. Organizing my feelings on paper is almost as cathartic for me as that afternoon chat was for Sam. Even better is having the privilege of bouncing my thoughts off all of you. And if your emails over the past 16 years are any indication, we're concerned about many of the same things. I hope you feel as reassured by that as I do.

Thanks for listening.

ACKNOWLEDGMENTS

To Helen, for helping me finish the final draft . . . and all the final drafts that followed.

To Becky and Rob, for being sources of inspiration and comfort to their proud father.

To Chris Barton, Tony Quinn, and the others at Fire Engineering Books & Videos, for the value they add to the publishing process.

To Hilary Gates and Jon Bassett, for their flexibility, professionalism, and good faith.

To Nancy Perry, who took a chance on an unconventional columnist and pointed me in the right direction more than once.

To Scott Cravens, for supporting strange ideas that could only come from a paramedic/writer/engineer/goaltender.

To Stan Fischler, for teaching a teenage hockey player to write for the fans.

To Bob Delagi, Eric Niegelberg, Ed Stapleton, and Paul Werfel: instructors, employers, mentors, and role models.

To my EMS partners, for being cool and careful during curious times. And to the men and women—even the New York Yankees fans—of Suffolk County Medical Control, for knowing when to follow and when to lead.

INDEX